COLOSTOMY DIET COOKBOOK FOR BEGINNERS

Nourishing Recipes and Expert Guidance for Optimal Health and Comfort After Surgery

Dr. Kelly Haaland

To show our appreciation for your purchase, we're delighted to offer you these special bonuses as a heartfelt thank you.

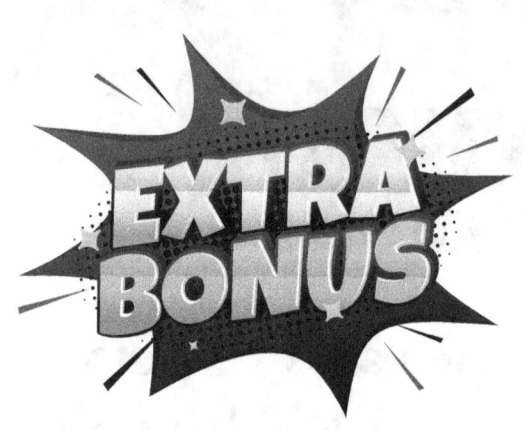 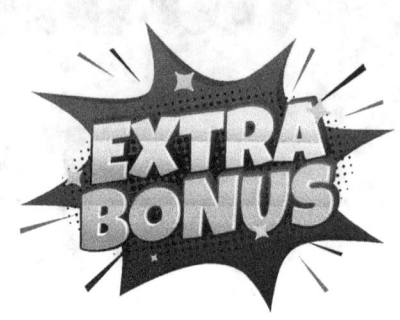

1. A Food Tracker Journal
2. Downloadable E-BOOK featuring full-color images of finished recipes
3. One-on-one consultation session with Dr. Kelly Haaland

Copyright © 2024 All rights reserved.

No part of this book may be reproduced or transmitted in any form or by any means, electronic or mechanical, including photocopying, recording, or by any information storage and retrieval system, without written permission from the author. The scanning, uploading, and distribution of this book via the internet or via any other means without the permission of the author is illegal and punishable by law. The author has made every effort to ensure the accuracy of the information contained in this book. However, the author cannot be held responsible for any errors or omissions.

Table of Contents

Introduction...7

Chapter 1
Understanding Colostomy..9
Basics of a Colostomy Diet...12
Foods to Include and Avoid..15
Essential Nutrients and Your Colostomy.....................18
Hydration and Colostomy...21

Breakfast
Banana Oatmeal..24
Scrambled Eggs...25
Avocado Toast...26
Mashed Potato Pancakes..27
Rice Porridge...28
Applesauce Pancakes..29
Poached Eggs..30
Cream of Wheat..31
Pumpkin Soup...32
Quinoa Porridge..33
Soft Baked Pear...34
Steamed Asparagus...35
Mild Vegetable Stir-Fry..36
Polenta...37
Ricotta Pancakes...38
Peach Compote...39
Baked Custard Oatmeal..40
Chia Seed Pudding...41
Rice Cakes with Avocado...42
Silken Tofu Smoothie...43

Poultry & Meat Recipes
Lamb Tagine..44
Pork Chop Puree...45

Chicken Tagine...46
Bison Meatballs..47
Grouper Fillets...48
Veal Paprikash...49
Beef Tenderloin...50
Pheasant Stew..51
Roast Turkey Breast..52
Chicken Porridge..53
Duck Confit..54
Braised Rabbit..55
Chicken Risotto..56
Soft-Cooked Chicken Thighs..57
Veal Scallopini..58
Lamb Puree..59
Turkey Patties..60
Oven-Poached Salmon...61
Beef Stew...62
Pulled Pork...63
Poached Chicken Breast..64

Vegetables
Fennel Puree..65
Bamboo Shoots..66
Watercress Soup..67
Stewed Tomatoes...68
Mushroom Broth...69
Turnip Soup..70
Celery Root Puree..71
Jicama Slaw...72
Kabocha Squash Soup...73
Plantain Porridge...74
Chayote Mash..75
Okra Stew..76
Sweet Corn Puree..77
Daikon Radish Salad..78
Roasted Parsnips...79
Asparagus Soup...80
Silken Tofu and Bok Choy..81
Beetroot Salad...82

Eggplant Dip..83
Pureed Peas..84
Zucchini Ribbons...85
Carrot Soup..86

Fish & Seafood Recipes
Shrimp and Rice Congee...87
Lingcod in Pesto..88
Monkfish Medallions..89
Squid Ink Pasta..90
Bouillabaisse..91
Sole Florentine..92
Snapper Veracruz..93
Barramundi with Lime...94
Catfish Creole..95
Oyster Stew..96
Salmon Mousse...97
Trout Almondine..98
Grouper Piccata..99
Sea Bass with Dill...100
Prawn Stir-Fry..101
Sautéed Calamari..102
Grilled Mahi-Mahi...103
Mussels Marinière..104
Lobster Bisque..105
Haddock Chowder...106
Tilapia in Parchment...107
Broiled Scallops..108
Flounder Meunière..109

Desserts
Zabaglione...110
Apple Crisp...111
Milky Semolina Pudding..112
Simple Poached Quince..113
Yogurt Parfait...114
Lemon Sponge Cake..115
Coconut Rice Pudding..116

Bread Pudding..117
Vanilla Panna Cotta..118

8-WEEK MEAL PLAN..119

BONUSES..130.

Dear Esteemed Reader

Each of us is as unique as the stories we carry, and this is especially true when it comes to our dietary needs. Our cookbook is designed to be a guide, a source of inspiration, and a companion in the kitchen for those seeking to maintain a healthy and balanced diet post-colostomy. However, it's important to remember that what works for one may not work for another. Just like a tailor adjusts a garment to fit its wearer perfectly, you may find that adjusting these recipes to suit your personal nutritional requirements and tastes is not only necessary but a delightful exploration of your preferences and needs.

We encourage you to consult with your healthcare provider or a dietitian as you make these adjustments. They can offer invaluable insights and guidance tailored specifically to you, ensuring that your diet supports your health and wellbeing in the best possible way.

Moreover, please bear in mind that the nutritional information provided with each recipe is an approximation. Factors such as the brand of ingredients used, portion sizes, and even the way your kitchen tools measure can influence the nutritional value of each dish. Therefore, view these numbers as a guide rather than an exact science, and feel free to make adjustments based on your nutritional goals and requirements.

Furthermore, If our cookbook has brought joy to your kitchen and table, we'd be thrilled to hear about your experiences in an Amazon review. On the flip side, if you stumble upon any hiccups while exploring our recipes, don't hesitate to get in touch at **kellyhaaland2@gmail.com** We're here to support your cooking journey every step of the way.

Introduction

Welcome to your new beginning! Whether you or a loved one has recently undergone a colostomy surgery, the journey you're embarking on is undoubtedly filled with a mix of emotions – apprehension, relief, and hope. It's a path that requires adjustments, not just physically but also in lifestyle, particularly in diet. That's where this book, "Colostomy Diet Cookbook for Beginners," comes into play, promising to be your compassionate companion as you navigate this new terrain. First things first: take a deep breath. You've made it through what is arguably the toughest part - the surgery. Now, you're faced with the challenge of adapting to your new normal, which includes making dietary choices that are crucial for your comfort and health. It might feel daunting at first, but guess what? You're not alone. This cookbook is designed to walk you through every step, ensuring that your transition is not just manageable but also enjoyable.

One might ask, why a special cookbook? Because after a colostomy, your body behaves differently. Certain foods that were once staples might now need to be eaten in moderation or prepared in a new way. But don't worry, this doesn't mean a lifetime of bland meals or long faces around the dinner table. Far from it! We're here to show you that post-colostomy eating can be full of delightful flavors, variety, and satisfaction. This cookbook is more than just a collection of recipes. It's a toolkit, a friend, and a roadmap. It's packed with easy-to-follow, delicious recipes that cater specifically to the post-colostomy diet, helping to manage symptoms and promote optimal healing. But it's also brimming with tips, tricks, and insights on how to live a full, vibrant life post-surgery.

We cover everything from how to handle social situations and dining out, to understanding how different foods can affect your body. Each recipe in this book has been carefully curated with your health and well-being in mind. They're not only nutritious and safe for a colostomy diet, but they're also mouthwateringly good – think of them as a culinary adventure, an opportunity to explore new tastes and textures, and maybe even discover a new favorite dish or two. Moreover, we understand that life doesn't slow down, and neither should you. That's why we've included a variety of quick, easy, and satisfying meals that fit perfectly into a busy lifestyle. Whether you're cooking for one or preparing a meal for the whole family, there's something here for everyone. Embracing this new chapter might feel a bit intimidating, but it's also filled with potential for growth, healing, and discovery. With this cookbook by your side, you'll find that your colostomy diet isn't a list of restrictions, but rather a new way to enjoy food while honoring your body's needs.

So, let's embark on this culinary journey together. With each page, you'll gain more confidence in your food choices, more joy in your meals, and a stronger sense of control over your health and well-being. Your colostomy may be a part of your life, but it doesn't define you. Here's to new beginnings, delicious meals, and a vibrant, healthy life ahead!

Chapter 1
Understanding Colostomy

Definition and Reasons for Colostomy
A colostomy is a surgical procedure that involves creating an opening in the abdominal wall through which the end of the colon (large intestine) is brought out. This opening, known as a stoma, serves as a new path for waste material to exit the body. The procedure is often necessitated by conditions that prevent the normal passage of stool through the rectum and anus. These conditions can include colorectal cancer, diverticulitis, inflammatory bowel disease (Crohn's disease or ulcerative colitis), trauma to the lower digestive tract, and congenital defects.

The Surgical Procedure
The colostomy surgery can be categorized as either temporary or permanent, depending on the underlying condition. The operation might involve removing a portion of the colon or rectum, with the remaining colon brought to the abdominal surface to form the stoma. This can be located anywhere on the abdomen, although it is commonly placed on the left-hand side.
There are various types of colostomies, named according to the part of the colon involved:
- **Ascending colostomy:** Rare and involves the ascending part of the colon.
- **Transverse colostomy:** Involves the transverse colon and is usually temporary.
- **Descending or sigmoid colostomy:** The most common type, involving the descending or sigmoid colon.

The surgery can be performed using traditional open surgery or minimally invasive techniques like laparoscopy, depending on the individual case and the surgeon's expertise.

Post-Surgery Recovery
Post-operative care is crucial for recovery and involves managing the stoma, ensuring proper healing, and preventing complications. Initially, patients may experience discomfort, and the stoma may be swollen, but it usually shrinks to its permanent size within a few

weeks. Learning how to care for the stoma and use colostomy bags is an essential part of the recovery process, often facilitated by stoma care nurses or specialists.

Living with a Colostomy

Adjusting to life after colostomy surgery can be challenging. It requires getting accustomed to the stoma and managing it daily, which includes tasks like emptying and changing the colostomy bag. Emotional and psychological support is also crucial, as individuals may go through a range of emotions, from relief of symptoms to anxiety or depression due to changes in body image and lifestyle.

Support groups and counseling can be beneficial, offering a platform to share experiences and coping strategies. Many find that, over time, they can return to most of their pre-surgery activities, including sports, travel, and work.

Diet and Nutrition

Diet plays a pivotal role in adapting to life with a colostomy. Initially, a special diet may be recommended to allow the bowel to heal and to prevent irritation of the stoma. Gradually, individuals can return to a more regular diet, although some may need to modify their intake to manage gas, odor, and stool consistency.

Hydration is particularly important, as the colon is responsible for water reabsorption, and its partial removal can affect fluid balance in the body. A balanced diet rich in vitamins, minerals, and fiber (when recommended) is essential, but dietary adjustments are often personalized, based on how the body reacts to different foods post-surgery.

Psychological Impact and Support

The psychological impact of undergoing colostomy can be significant. Individuals may experience feelings of self-consciousness, anxiety, or depression due to the change in their body function and self-image. Professional counseling, support groups, and connecting with others who have undergone similar experiences can be incredibly beneficial. These resources offer emotional support, practical tips, and encouragement, helping individuals navigate the challenges and lead fulfilling lives post-surgery.

Long-Term Management
Long-term management of a colostomy involves routine care of the stoma, monitoring for any signs of complications (such as infection, skin irritation, or herniation), and regular medical check-ups. Maintaining a healthy lifestyle, including a balanced diet, regular exercise, and avoiding activities that might strain the abdominal area, is crucial.
With advancements in medical supplies, colostomy bags have become more user-friendly, discreet, and comfortable, enabling individuals to lead active, normal lives. Many find they can engage in sports, travel, and other activities they enjoyed before surgery.

Hence, understanding colostomy is vital for those who are about to undergo the procedure, their loved ones, and anyone interested in learning about this aspect of healthcare. It's a significant adjustment that involves changes in body function, self-care routines, and lifestyle. However, with the right information, support, and care, individuals with a colostomy can lead healthy, active lives. It's important to focus on the positives, such as the relief of painful symptoms and the prevention of more severe health issues, which the surgery often provides. Embracing the new normal with confidence and optimism is key to adapting successfully to life post-colostomy.

Basics of a Colostomy Diet

The basics of a colostomy diet are crucial for individuals who have undergone a colostomy surgery to understand and implement. This diet is designed to help manage the output of the stoma, prevent complications, and ensure that the individual maintains proper nutrition. The transition to this specialized diet can be challenging, but with the right knowledge and guidance, individuals can lead healthy and comfortable lives. After a colostomy, the body's way of processing food changes, which necessitates adjustments in eating habits. The diet aims to minimize issues like gas, odor, diarrhea, and constipation, ensuring the stoma functions correctly and comfortably. It's not about strict limitations but rather about finding what works best for the individual's specific situation.

Initial Post-Surgery Diet
Immediately following surgery, the diet is typically liquid, transitioning slowly to include low-fiber foods. This gradual progression allows the bowel to heal and helps the individual adjust to the new digestive system functionality. Foods are reintroduced step by step, monitoring how the body reacts to different types of food.

Long-Term Dietary Adjustments
Once healed, most individuals can return to a normal diet but with heightened awareness of how certain foods affect their stoma output. Here are key components and considerations for a balanced colostomy diet:

Fiber Intake
- Gradual Fiber Introduction: After the initial healing period, fiber is reintroduced slowly. Some people may need to limit high-fiber foods to prevent blockages, while others find they can tolerate a regular fiber intake.
- Monitor Effects: Individual responses to fiber can vary, so it's important to monitor how different foods affect stoma output and consistency.

Fluids and Hydration
- **Stay Hydrated:** Adequate fluid intake is essential, especially since the colon plays a significant role in water reabsorption. Drinking plenty of water helps prevent dehydration and ensures proper stoma function.
- **Balance Electrolytes:** Maintaining a balance of electrolytes is crucial, as the altered colon function can sometimes lead to imbalances.

Managing Gas and Odor
- **Identify Trigger Foods:** Certain foods like onions, garlic, broccoli, and beans can cause gas or odors. Keeping a food diary helps identify personal triggers.
- **Moderation is Key:** It might not be necessary to completely eliminate gas-producing foods, but moderating their intake can help manage symptoms.

Food Preparation and Consumption
- **Chew Well:** Chewing food thoroughly is essential to break down food particles, aiding digestion and preventing blockages at the stoma site.
- **Meal Frequency:** Smaller, more frequent meals can be easier on the digestive system than large, heavy meals.

Special Considerations
- **Avoid Blockages:** Foods that can cause blockages, such as nuts, seeds, popcorn, and certain raw vegetables, should be consumed with caution or avoided based on individual tolerance.
- **Vitamin and Mineral Absorption:** Some individuals may face challenges with nutrient absorption, especially if significant portions of the intestine have been removed. Supplements may be necessary based on a healthcare provider's advice.

Monitoring and Adjusting the Diet

Adapting to a colostomy diet is a personal journey, and what works for one person may not work for another. Regular monitoring and adjusting of the diet are essential to find a balance that suits the individual's lifestyle and stoma output. Consulting with a dietitian who has experience with colostomy diets can be incredibly beneficial in creating a personalized eating plan.

Emotional and Psychological Considerations
Adjusting to the dietary changes post-colostomy can also have emotional and psychological impacts. Acceptance and patience are key, as is seeking support from healthcare providers, support groups, or counselors who understand the challenges of living with a colostomy.

In summary, the basics of a colostomy diet revolve around understanding how different foods affect the stoma, maintaining proper nutrition, and preventing complications. It's about making informed choices, closely monitoring how the body responds, and adjusting as necessary to find a diet that supports a healthy and active lifestyle. With careful management, most individuals with a colostomy can enjoy a diverse and satisfying diet while effectively managing their stoma.

Foods to Include and Avoid

Navigating the dietary landscape with a colostomy involves understanding which foods to include for optimal health and which to avoid to prevent discomfort or complications. This thorough analysis will focus on the foods that are generally recommended and those that are typically advised against for individuals with a colostomy, keeping in mind that personal tolerance can vary widely.

Foods to Include

Easy-to-Digest Vegetables and Fruits
- **Cooked Vegetables:** Soft, cooked vegetables like carrots, spinach, and squash are usually well-tolerated and provide essential nutrients.
- **Skinless Fruits:** Apples, pears, and peaches without skins can be easier to digest and less likely to cause blockages.

Lean Proteins
- **Meats and Poultry:** Well-cooked, tender cuts of meat and poultry can be included in the diet. They should be chewed thoroughly to aid in digestion.
- **Fish:** Offers a high-quality protein source that's typically easy to digest and provides omega-3 fatty acids.

Grains and Starches
- **Refined Grains:** White bread, pasta, and white rice are generally well-tolerated and less likely to cause issues than their whole-grain counterparts.
- **Potatoes:** Well-cooked and without skins, potatoes are a good source of energy and nutrients.

Dairy or Alternatives
- **Low-Lactose Options:** If lactose intolerance is not an issue, small amounts of dairy can be included. Otherwise, lactose-free alternatives or well-tolerated fermented dairy like yogurt can be beneficial.

Hydration
- **Water and Fluids**: Adequate hydration is crucial; water, herbal teas, and other non-caffeinated, non-alcoholic beverages are good choices.

Foods to Avoid or Limit
High-Fiber Foods
- **Raw Vegetables**: Especially those with skins, seeds, or tough stalks, as they can cause blockages or gas.
- **Whole Grains**: Foods like whole grain bread, brown rice, and quinoa might be too harsh initially and should be reintroduced slowly and monitored for tolerance.

Gas-Producing Foods
- **Certain Vegetables**: Onions, cabbage, beans, and broccoli are known to produce gas and might cause discomfort or distention.
- **Carbonated Beverages**: Soda and sparkling water can increase gas and bloating.

Odor-Producing Foods
- **Certain Fish and Meats**: Some types of seafood and red meats might increase stool odor.
- **Garlic and Spices**: These can cause odor issues for some individuals and might need to be limited.

High-Fat and Fried Foods
- **Greasy or Fried Items**: These can be harder to digest and may cause loose stools or discomfort.
- **Rich Desserts**: Foods high in fat and sugar can exacerbate digestive issues.

Foods with Hulls or Seeds
- **Nuts and Seeds**: These can be difficult to digest completely and pose a risk for blockage.
- **Popcorn**: It's often recommended to avoid popcorn due to its indigestible hulls, which can cause obstructions.

Monitoring and Personalization
The key to managing a colostomy diet effectively is personalization. Individuals are encouraged to keep a food diary to track what they eat and note any symptoms or changes in stoma output. This record can help identify specific foods that cause issues and those that are well-tolerated.

Gradual reintroduction of foods and careful monitoring is essential. Starting with small portions and slowly increasing them while observing the body's response can help in determining what is safe to consume regularly.

Consultation with Healthcare Providers
It's crucial for individuals with a colostomy to work closely with their healthcare team, including a dietitian, to develop a diet plan that meets their nutritional needs while accommodating their colostomy. They can provide guidance on how to introduce new foods, adjust the diet as needed, and ensure that the individual is maintaining proper nutrition.

Managing a diet with a colostomy involves a balance of including nutrient-dense foods that support overall health while avoiding those that might cause discomfort, gas, odor, or blockages. It's a highly individualized process, with personal tolerance dictating much of what can be included or should be avoided. With careful monitoring, most individuals with a colostomy can enjoy a varied and satisfying diet, maintaining their health and well-being post-surgery.

Essential Nutrients and Your Colostomy

Understanding the essential nutrients and their role in managing a colostomy is vital for anyone who has undergone this surgical procedure. The body's nutrient needs might change post-colostomy, and adapting to these changes is crucial for maintaining overall health and ensuring the stoma functions properly.

Macronutrients

Proteins
- Importance: Proteins are crucial for healing post-surgery, maintaining muscle mass, and supporting immune function. They are vital for tissue repair, especially important in the early stages after colostomy surgery.
- Sources: Include lean meats, poultry, fish, eggs, dairy products, and plant-based proteins like legumes, soy products, and nuts. Ensuring a high-quality protein intake can aid in recovery and stoma health.

Carbohydrates
- Importance: Carbohydrates are the body's primary energy source, essential for fueling all bodily functions and aiding in the healing process.
- Sources: Focus on easily digestible carbohydrates like white bread, rice, pasta, and certain cooked fruits and vegetables initially. Gradually, more fiber-containing foods can be reintroduced, monitoring for any changes in stoma output or discomfort.

Fats
- Importance: Fats are crucial for nutrient absorption, particularly for fat-soluble vitamins (A, D, E, K), and are important for cellular health.
- Sources: Incorporate healthy fats from avocados, olive oil, nuts, and seeds. However, it's essential to moderate fat intake, as excessive amounts can cause loose stools or increase the risk of heart disease.

Micronutrients
Vitamins and Minerals
- **Importance**: Essential for overall health, supporting immune function, bone health, and wound healing. Special attention should be paid to vitamins A, C, D, E, and K, along with minerals like iron, calcium, and zinc.
- **Sources**: A well-balanced diet including a variety of fruits, vegetables, whole grains, and lean proteins can provide these nutrients. However, some individuals may need supplementation, especially if they have absorption issues or dietary restrictions.

Fluids and Electrolytes
- **Importance**: Maintaining hydration is crucial, as the colon plays a significant role in water reabsorption. Electrolytes like sodium, potassium, and chloride are vital for fluid balance and nerve and muscle function.
- **Sources**: Adequate intake of water, herbal teas, and other non-caffeinated beverages is recommended. Foods rich in potassium and sodium, like bananas, potatoes, and broth, can help maintain electrolyte balance.

Fiber
- **Importance**: Fiber is essential for bowel function and can help manage stoma output consistency. However, the amount and type of fiber can vary based on individual tolerance.
- **Sources**: Initially, low-residue foods are recommended post-surgery. Gradually, soluble fiber sources like oatmeal, ripe bananas, and applesauce can be introduced, followed by more fibrous foods as tolerated.

Special Nutritional Considerations
- **Vitamin B12 Absorption**: Depending on the portion of the bowel affected or removed, vitamin B12 absorption might be compromised, necessitating supplementation.
- **Iron Absorption**: Iron deficiency can be a concern, especially if parts of the colon or ileum are removed, affecting iron absorption. Monitoring and supplementation might be necessary.

- **Calcium and Vitamin D**: Important for bone health, especially if steroid medications are used or if there's a risk of osteoporosis.

Monitoring and Adjusting Your Diet
Regular follow-ups with healthcare providers, including a dietitian, are essential for ongoing monitoring of nutritional status and stoma health. Nutritional needs can change over time, and adapting the diet to meet these changing requirements is crucial. Keeping a food and symptom diary can help identify any foods or nutrients that may need adjustment.

Hence, nutrition plays a pivotal role in the life of someone with a colostomy. Understanding and managing the intake of essential nutrients is crucial for maintaining health, ensuring proper stoma function, and enhancing quality of life. Individual needs can vary significantly, making personalized dietary advice and regular medical monitoring key components of successful colostomy management. With the right nutritional care, individuals with a colostomy can lead healthy, active lives.

Hydration and Colostomy

Hydration plays a pivotal role in the overall health and well-being of individuals with a colostomy. The colon, part of the large intestine, is primarily responsible for water reabsorption in the digestive system. When a section of the colon is bypassed or removed, it can significantly impact fluid balance in the body. Understanding the intricacies of hydration is crucial for those living with a colostomy to maintain optimal health, prevent complications, and ensure the stoma functions properly.

The Importance of Hydration
Hydration is crucial for several physiological functions, including:
- Digestive health: Adequate fluid intake helps in maintaining the right consistency of stoma output, preventing issues like constipation or thickened stool, which can lead to blockages.
- Nutrient absorption: Water plays a vital role in dissolving nutrients so they can be absorbed efficiently by the body.
- Detoxification: Adequate hydration aids in flushing out waste products and toxins from the body.
- Body temperature regulation: Fluids help in maintaining body temperature through sweat and respiration.
- Skin integrity: Proper hydration is essential for maintaining healthy skin around the stoma site.

Challenges in Maintaining Hydration
Individuals with a colostomy might face specific challenges in staying hydrated:
- **Altered Water Reabsorption:** Since the colon is crucial for water reabsorption, a colostomy can disrupt this balance, leading to an increased risk of dehydration.
- **Stoma Output Management:** The consistency and volume of stoma output can vary, and high output levels can lead to fluid loss.
- **Dietary Changes:** Adjustments in diet, particularly if fluid-rich foods are reduced, can impact hydration status.

Strategies for Effective Hydration
Maintaining optimal hydration requires mindful strategies:
- **Adequate Fluid Intake:** It's generally recommended to drink at least 8 cups (about 2 liters) of fluid daily, but needs can vary based on individual factors, including climate, activity level, and stoma output.
- **Monitoring Fluid Output:** Keeping an eye on the amount and consistency of stoma output can provide insights into hydration status. High output, particularly if it's watery, can indicate a need for increased fluid intake.
- **Balanced Electrolyte Intake:** Electrolytes like sodium, potassium, and chloride are essential for fluid balance and nerve and muscle function. Incorporating a balanced intake of electrolytes, especially if there is significant stoma output, is crucial.
- **Recognizing Signs of Dehydration:** Symptoms can include dry mouth, thirst, reduced urine output, dark-colored urine, fatigue, dizziness, and headache. Promptly addressing these signs is important to prevent complications.

Fluid Choices and Considerations
- **Water:** The cornerstone of hydration, plain water is usually the best option. It's calorie-free, sugar-free, and readily available.
- **Other Fluids:** Herbal teas, clear broths, and electrolyte solutions can also contribute to fluid intake. Caffeinated beverages and alcohol should be consumed in moderation as they can have a diuretic effect.
- **Fluid-Rich Foods:** Foods like soups, fruits, and vegetables can contribute to overall fluid intake and provide additional nutrients.

Special Considerations
- **High Stoma Output:** Individuals experiencing high stoma output should be particularly vigilant about their fluid intake to counterbalance the loss of water and electrolytes.
- **Hot Weather and Physical Activity:** These conditions can increase fluid requirements. Adjusting intake accordingly is necessary to prevent dehydration.

- **Illness:** Conditions like diarrhea or vomiting can lead to rapid fluid loss, necessitating increased fluid intake or even medical intervention to prevent dehydration.

Collaboration with Healthcare Providers

Regular consultations with healthcare providers, including a gastroenterologist, stoma nurse, or dietitian, are vital. They can offer personalized advice, help monitor hydration status, and adjust dietary or fluid recommendations based on individual needs and the specifics of the stoma output.

BREAKFAST RECIPES

1. Banana Oatmeal
Ingredients:
- 1 ripe banana, mashed
- 1 cup rolled oats
- 2 cups water or milk (for a creamier texture)
- Pinch of salt
- ½ teaspoon cinnamon (optional)
- 1 tablespoon honey or maple syrup (optional)

Instructions:
1. In a medium saucepan, combine the oats, water/milk, mashed banana, and a pinch of salt.
2. Bring the mixture to a boil, then reduce the heat to low.
3. Simmer for 5-10 minutes, stirring occasionally, until the oats are soft and have absorbed the liquid.
4. Remove from heat and stir in cinnamon and honey/maple syrup if using.
5. Serve hot.

Servings: 2
Nutritional Information (per serving, without optional ingredients):
- Calories: 307
- Protein: 11g
- Carbohydrates: 56g
- Fat: 5g
- Fiber: 8g
- Sugar: 7g

Cooking Time: 15 minutes

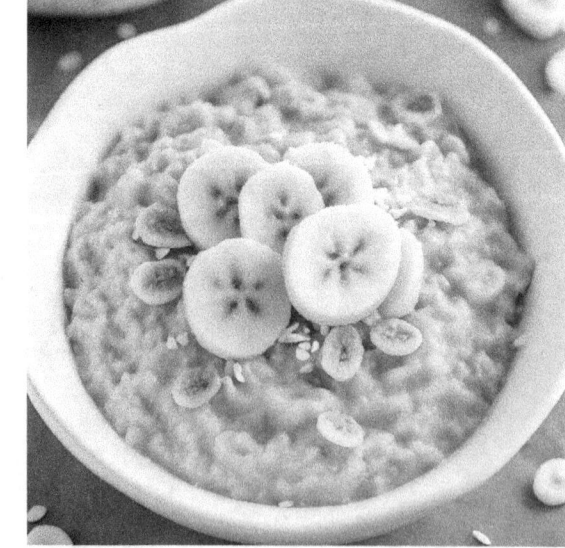

2. Scrambled Eggs

Ingredients:
- 4 large eggs
- 2 tablespoons milk or water
- Salt and pepper to taste
- 1 tablespoon butter or oil

Instructions:
1. In a bowl, whisk together the eggs, milk/water, salt, and pepper.
2. Heat butter/oil in a non-stick skillet over medium heat.
3. Pour in the egg mixture. As the eggs begin to set, gently pull the eggs across the pan with a spatula, forming large soft curds.
4. Continue cooking – pulling, lifting, and folding eggs – until thickened and no visible liquid egg remains. Do not stir constantly.
5. Remove from the heat when the eggs are cooked but still slightly moist.

Servings: 2

Nutritional Information (per serving):
- Calories: 215
- Protein: 14g
- Carbohydrates: 2g
- Fat: 16g
- Cholesterol: 372mg
- Sodium: 189mg

Cooking Time: 10 minutes

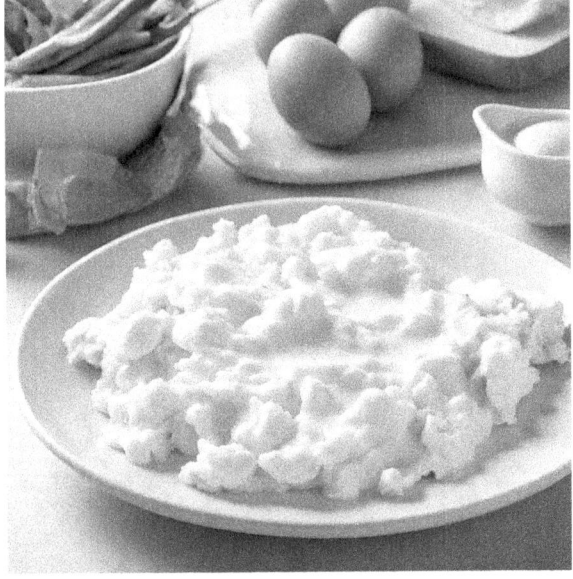

3. Avocado Toast

Ingredients:
- 2 slices whole grain bread
- 1 ripe avocado
- Salt and pepper to taste
- Lemon juice (optional)

Instructions:
1. Toast the bread slices to your preferred doneness.
2. Halve the avocado, remove the pit, and scoop out the flesh into a bowl.
3. Mash the avocado with a fork and season with salt, pepper, and a few drops of lemon juice if desired.
4. Spread the mashed avocado evenly onto the toasted bread slices.

Servings: 2

Nutritional Information (per serving):
- Calories: 237
- Protein: 5g
- Carbohydrates: 26g
- Fat: 14g
- Fiber: 10g
- Sugar: 3g

Cooking Time: 5 minutes

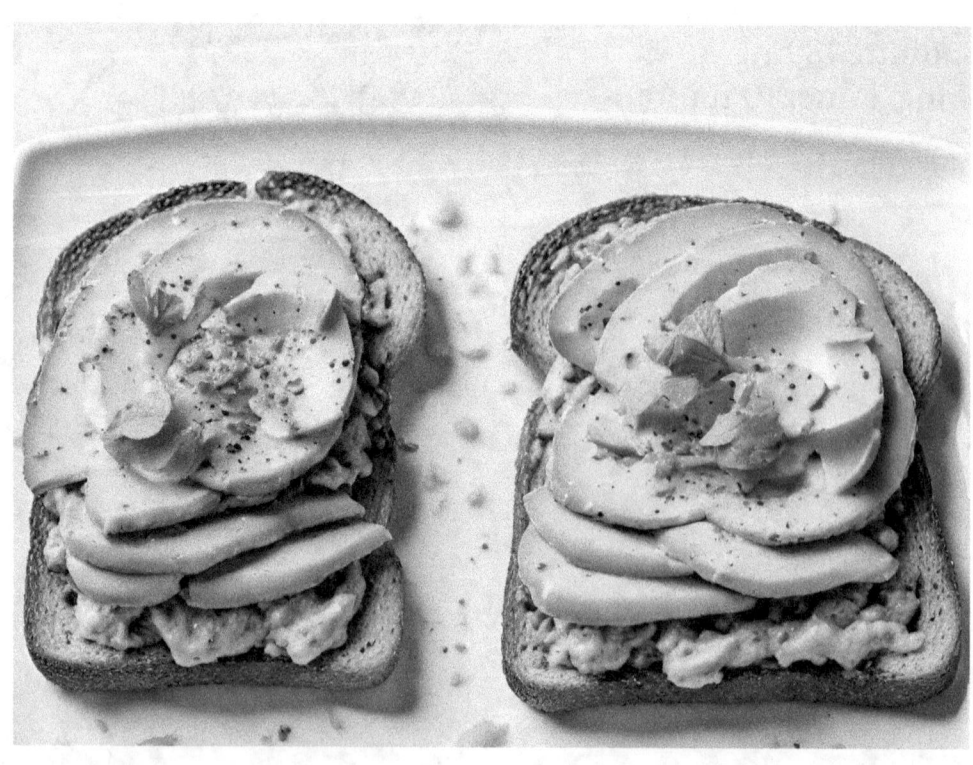

4. Mashed Potato Pancakes

Ingredients:
- 2 cups mashed potatoes (cooled)
- 1 large egg, beaten
- ¼ cup all-purpose flour (or more, as needed)
- Salt and pepper to taste
- 2 tablespoons olive oil or butter for frying

Instructions:
1. In a large bowl, combine the mashed potatoes, beaten egg, flour, salt, and pepper. Stir until well combined. If the mixture is too sticky, add a bit more flour.
2. Heat oil/butter in a large skillet over medium heat.
3. Form the potato mixture into patties and fry until golden brown on both sides, about 3-4 minutes per side.
4. Transfer to a paper towel-lined plate to drain any excess oil.

Servings: 4 pancakes

Nutritional Information (per pancake):
- Calories: 209
- Protein: 4g
- Carbohydrates: 28g
- Fat: 9g
- Fiber: 2g
- Sugar: 1g

Cooking Time: 20 minutes

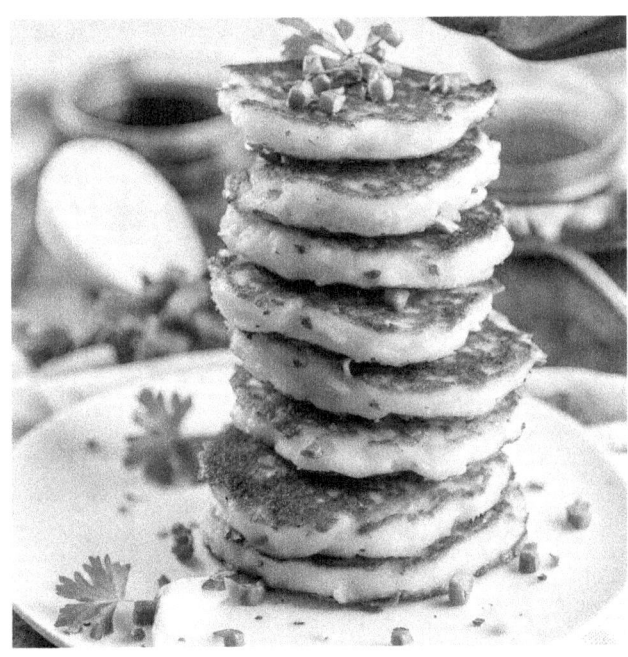

5. Rice Porridge

Ingredients:
- 1 cup white rice
- 4 cups water or broth
- Pinch of salt

Instructions:
1. Rinse the rice under cold water until the water runs clear.
2. In a large pot, combine the rice, water/broth, and salt.
3. Bring to a boil, then reduce the heat to low, cover, and simmer for about 30 minutes, stirring occasionally, until the rice is soft and the porridge has a creamy consistency.
4. Serve warm, adding more water or broth if a thinner consistency is desired.

Servings: 4

Nutritional Information (per serving):
- Calories: 169
- Protein: 3g
- Carbohydrates: 37g
- Fat: 0.3g
- Fiber: 0.6g
- Sugar: 0g

Cooking Time: 30 minutes

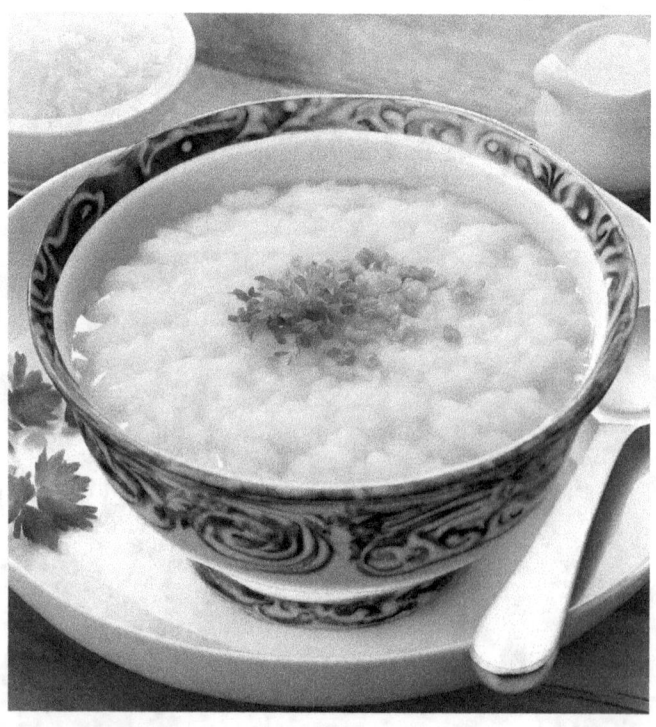

6. Applesauce Pancakes

Ingredients:
- 1 cup all-purpose flour
- 1 tablespoon sugar
- 1 teaspoon baking powder
- ½ teaspoon baking soda
- ¼ teaspoon salt
- 1 cup unsweetened applesauce
- ½ cup milk
- 2 tablespoons melted butter
- 1 egg

Instructions:
1. In a large bowl, whisk together the flour, sugar, baking powder, baking soda, and salt.
2. In another bowl, combine the applesauce, milk, melted butter, and egg.
3. Pour the wet ingredients into the dry ingredients and stir until just combined.
4. Heat a non-stick skillet over medium heat and pour ¼ cup batter for each pancake.
5. Cook until bubbles form on the surface, then flip and cook until golden brown.

Servings: 4

Nutritional Information (per serving):
- Calories: 224
- Protein: 6g
- Carbohydrates: 39g
- Fat: 5g
- Fiber: 2g
- Sugar: 11g

Cooking Time: 20 minutes

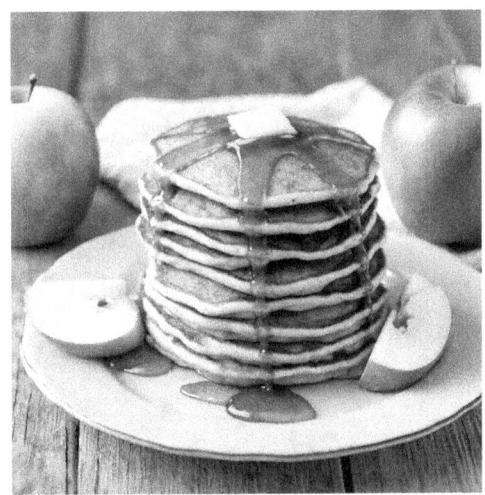

7. Poached Eggs

Ingredients:
- 4 large eggs
- Water for poaching
- 1 teaspoon vinegar (optional)

Instructions:
1. Fill a saucepan with 3 inches of water, add vinegar, and bring to a simmer.
2. Crack each egg into a small bowl and gently slide it into the simmering water.
3. Cook for 3-4 minutes until the whites are set but the yolks are still runny.
4. Use a slotted spoon to remove the eggs and drain on a kitchen towel.

Servings: 4

Nutritional Information (per egg):
- Calories: 68
- Protein: 6g
- Carbohydrates: 0.6g
- Fat: 4.7g
- Cholesterol: 186mg
- Sodium: 70mg

Cooking Time: 10 minutes

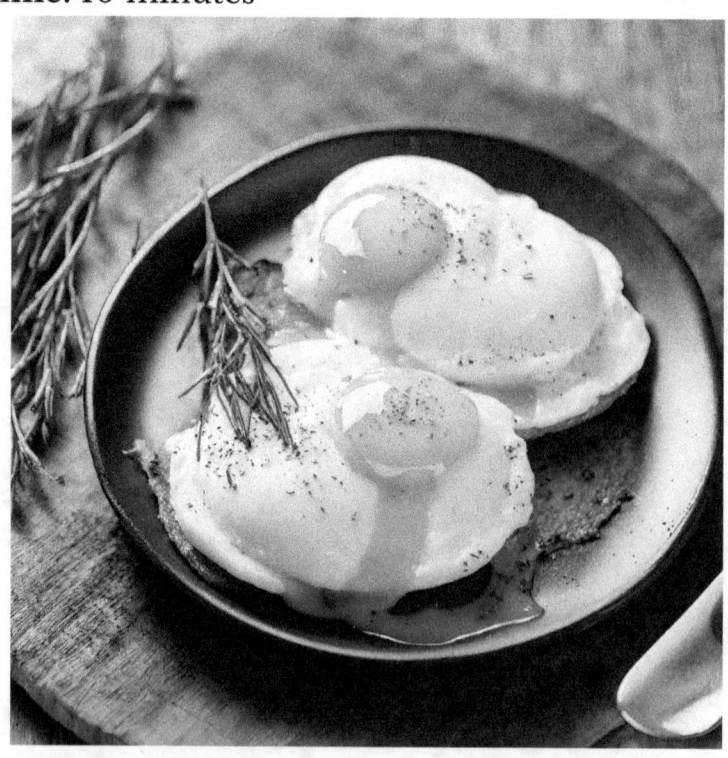

8. Cream of Wheat

Ingredients:
- 1 cup cream of wheat (farina)
- 4 cups water or milk
- Pinch of salt
- Sweetener or spices (optional, to taste)

Instructions:
1. Bring water or milk to a boil in a saucepan. Add a pinch of salt.
2. Gradually whisk in the cream of wheat, reduce the heat to low, and cook for 2-3 minutes, stirring constantly, until thickened.
3. Remove from heat and add sweetener or spices if desired.

Servings: 4

Nutritional Information (per serving):
- Calories: 150 (with water)
- Protein: 5g
- Carbohydrates: 31g
- Fat: 0.5g
- Fiber: 1g
- Sugar: 0g (without added sweetener)

Cooking Time: 10 minutes

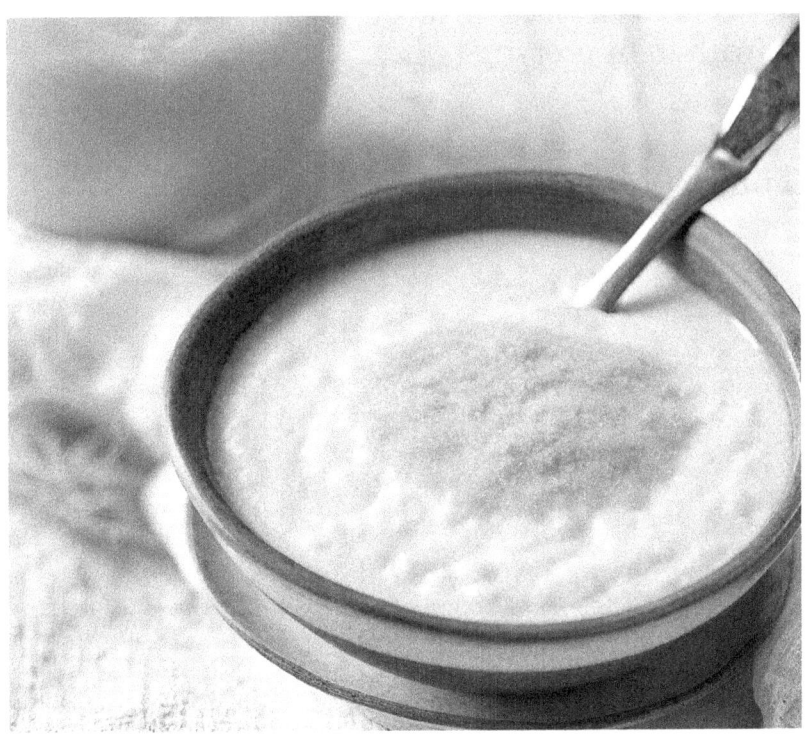

9. Pumpkin Soup

Ingredients:
- 2 cups pumpkin puree (canned or fresh)
- 3 cups vegetable broth
- 1 onion, finely chopped
- 1 clove garlic, minced
- 1 cup light cream or coconut milk
- Salt and pepper to taste
- 1 tablespoon olive oil

Instructions:
1. Heat olive oil in a large pot over medium heat. Add onion and garlic, sautéing until soft.
2. Add pumpkin puree and vegetable broth, bring to a boil, then reduce heat and simmer for 20 minutes.
3. Puree the soup with an immersion blender or in batches with a regular blender until smooth.
4. Stir in the cream or coconut milk, and season with salt and pepper. Heat through without boiling.

Servings: 4

Nutritional Information (per serving):
- Calories: 180
- Protein: 2g
- Carbohydrates: 18g
- Fat: 12g (with light cream)
- Fiber: 5g
- Sugar: 8g

Cooking Time: 30 minutes

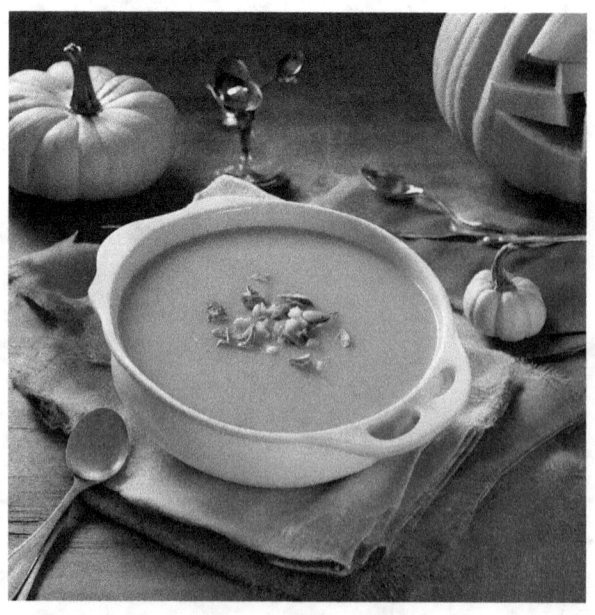

10. Quinoa Porridge

Ingredients:
- 1 cup quinoa, rinsed
- 2 cups water or milk
- 1/2 teaspoon cinnamon
- 1 tablespoon honey or maple syrup (optional)
- Fresh fruit or nuts for topping (optional)

Instructions:
1. Combine quinoa and water/milk in a saucepan and bring to a boil.
2. Reduce heat to low, cover, and simmer for 15 minutes or until liquid is absorbed.
3. Stir in cinnamon and sweetener if using.
4. Serve warm, topped with fresh fruit or nuts if desired.

Servings: 4

Nutritional Information (per serving):
- Calories: 222
- Protein: 8g
- Carbohydrates: 39g
- Fat: 3.5g
- Fiber: 4g
- Sugar: 0g (without added sweeteners)

Cooking Time: 20 minutes

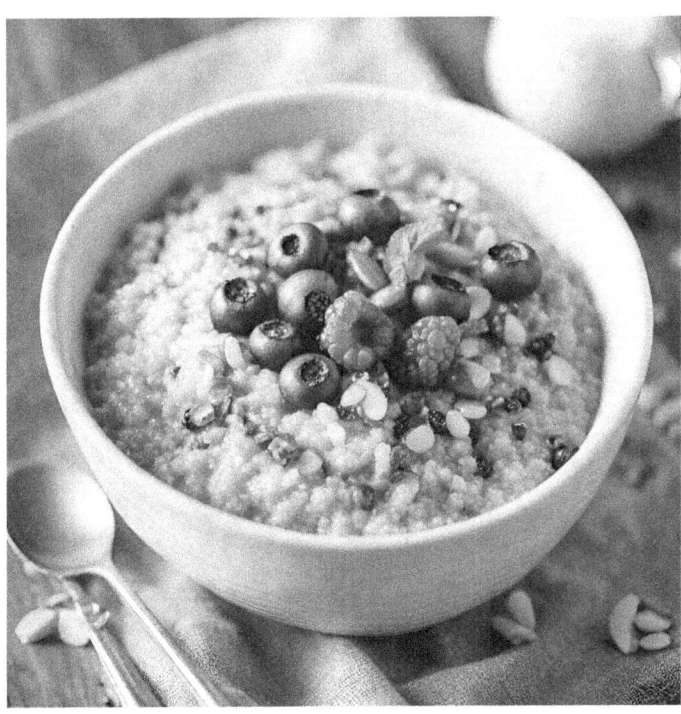

11. Soft Baked Pear

Ingredients:
- 4 ripe pears, halved and cored
- 2 tablespoons honey or maple syrup
- 1/2 teaspoon cinnamon
- 1/4 cup walnuts, chopped (optional)

Instructions:
1. Preheat the oven to 350°F (175°C).
2. Place the pear halves on a baking dish, cut-side up.
3. Drizzle with honey or maple syrup and sprinkle with cinnamon.
4. Bake for 20-25 minutes or until pears are soft and slightly caramelized.
5. Serve warm, sprinkled with chopped walnuts if desired.

Servings: 4

Nutritional Information (per serving, without walnuts):
- Calories: 150
- Protein: 1g
- Carbohydrates: 36g
- Fat: 0.2g
- Fiber: 6g
- Sugar: 28g

Cooking Time: 30 minutes

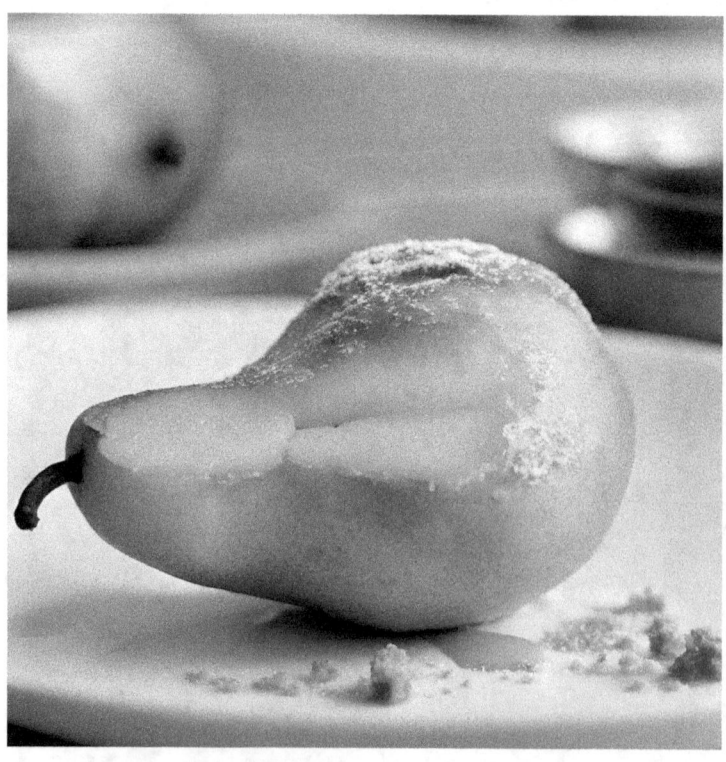

12. Steamed Asparagus

Ingredients:
- 1 pound asparagus, trimmed
- Salt and pepper to taste
- Lemon wedges for serving (optional)

Instructions:
1. Fill a pot with enough water to reach the bottom of the steamer basket and bring to a boil.
2. Place asparagus in the steamer basket and steam for 3-5 minutes, until tender but still slightly crisp.
3. Remove from heat, season with salt and pepper, and serve with lemon wedges if desired.

Servings: 4

Nutritional Information (per serving):
- Calories: 27
- Protein: 3g
- Carbohydrates: 5g
- Fat: 0.2g
- Fiber: 2.8g
- Sugar: 2.5g

Cooking Time: 10 minutes

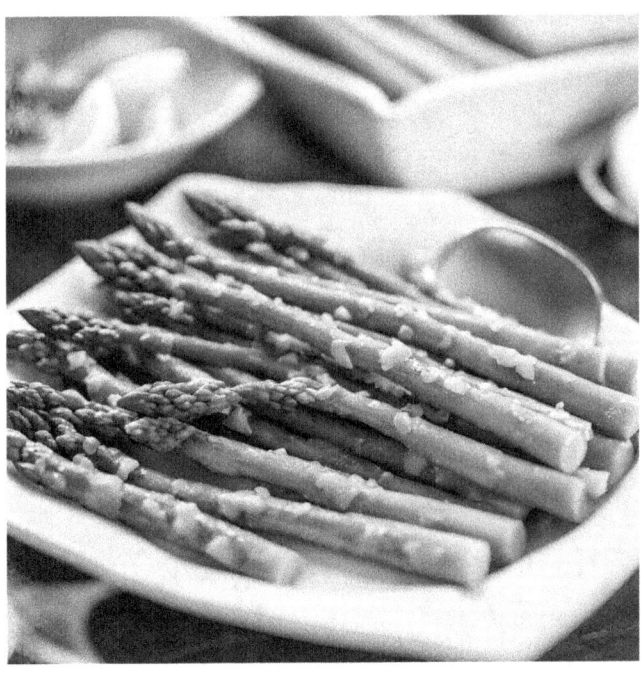

13. Mild Vegetable Stir-Fry

Ingredients:
- 2 cups mixed vegetables (e.g., carrots, bell peppers, zucchini), thinly sliced
- 1 tablespoon olive oil
- 2 cloves garlic, minced
- 1 tablespoon soy sauce (or to taste)
- Salt and pepper to taste

Instructions:
1. Heat olive oil in a large skillet or wok over medium-high heat.
2. Add the garlic and sauté for 30 seconds.
3. Add the mixed vegetables and stir-fry for 5-7 minutes or until vegetables are tender-crisp.
4. Stir in soy sauce, and season with salt and pepper to taste.

Servings: 4

Nutritional Information (per serving):
- Calories: 80
- Protein: 2g
- Carbohydrates: 10g
- Fat: 4g
- Fiber: 3g
- Sugar: 5g

Cooking Time: 15 minutes

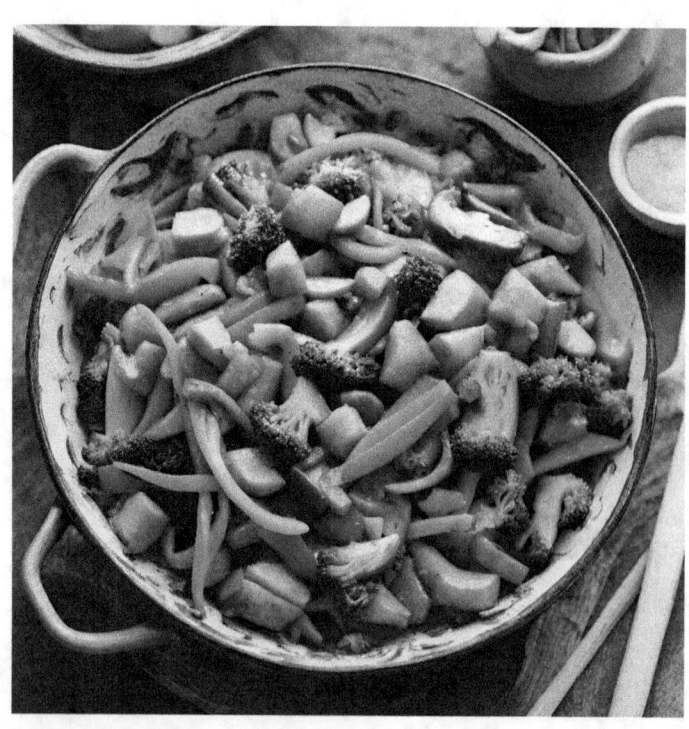

14. Polenta

Ingredients:
- 1 cup polenta (cornmeal)
- 4 cups water or broth
- 1 teaspoon salt
- 2 tablespoons butter (optional)
- 1/4 cup grated Parmesan cheese (optional)

Instructions:
1. Bring water or broth to a boil in a large saucepan. Add salt.
2. Gradually whisk in the polenta. Reduce heat to low and cook, stirring often, until the mixture thickens and the polenta is tender, about 30-40 minutes.
3. Remove from heat and optionally stir in butter and Parmesan cheese until well incorporated.
4. Serve warm or spread onto a flat surface to cool and solidify, then cut into squares.

Servings: 4

Nutritional Information (per serving, without optional ingredients):
- Calories: 150
- Protein: 3g
- Carbohydrates: 32g
- Fat: 1g
- Fiber: 2g
- Sugar: 0g

Cooking Time: 40-50 minutes

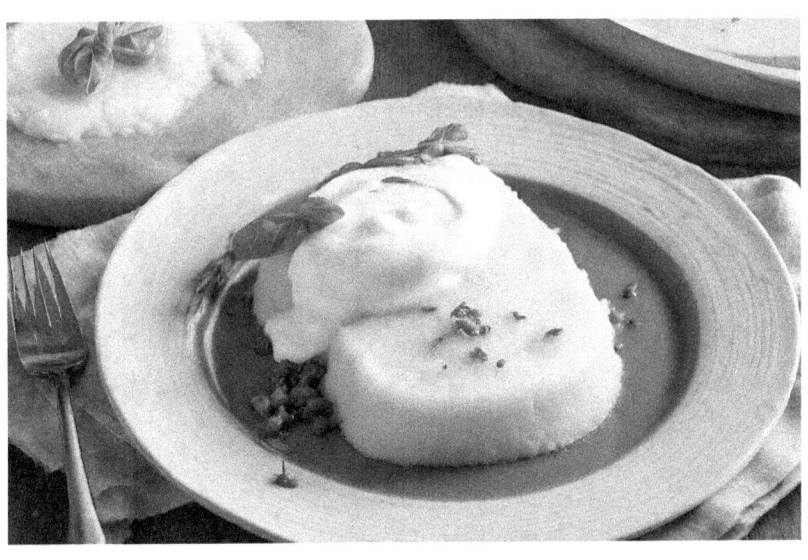

15. Ricotta Pancakes

Ingredients:
- 1 cup all-purpose flour
- 2 tablespoons sugar
- 1 teaspoon baking powder
- 1/2 teaspoon baking soda
- 1/4 teaspoon salt
- 3/4 cup ricotta cheese
- 1/2 cup milk
- 2 large eggs
- 1/2 teaspoon vanilla extract

Instructions:
1. In a large bowl, combine flour, sugar, baking powder, baking soda, and salt.
2. In another bowl, whisk together ricotta, milk, eggs, and vanilla.
3. Fold the wet ingredients into the dry ingredients until just combined.
4. Heat a non-stick skillet over medium heat and spoon 1/4 cup of batter for each pancake.
5. Cook until bubbles form on the surface, then flip and cook until golden brown.

Servings: 4

Nutritional Information (per serving):
- Calories: 280
- Protein: 14g
- Carbohydrates: 35g
- Fat: 9g
- Fiber: 1g
- Sugar: 8g

Cooking Time: 20 minutes

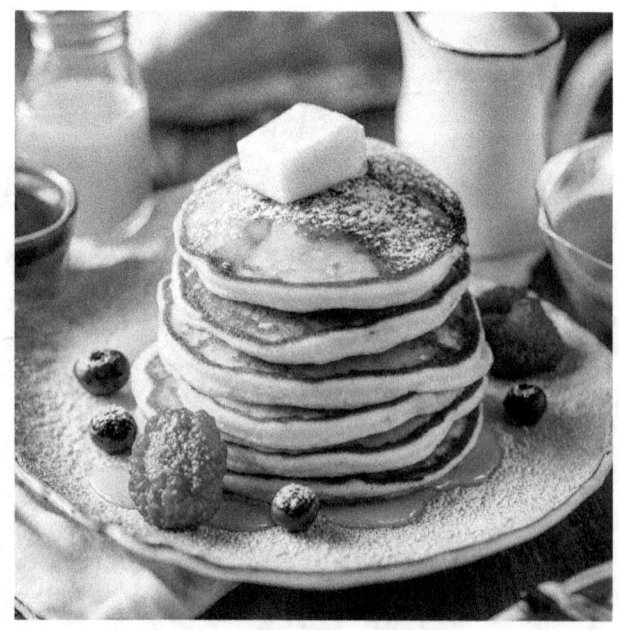

16. Peach Compote

Ingredients:
- 4 ripe peaches, peeled, pitted, and sliced
- 1/4 cup sugar or honey
- 1/2 teaspoon cinnamon
- 1/4 cup water

Instructions:
1. Combine peaches, sugar/honey, cinnamon, and water in a saucepan.
2. Bring to a simmer over medium heat, stirring occasionally.
3. Cook for 10-15 minutes or until the peaches are soft and the sauce has thickened slightly.
4. Let cool slightly and serve warm or chilled.

Servings: 4

Nutritional Information (per serving):
- Calories: 120
- Protein: 1g
- Carbohydrates: 31g
- Fat: 0.2g
- Fiber: 2g
- Sugar: 29g

Cooking Time: 20 minutes

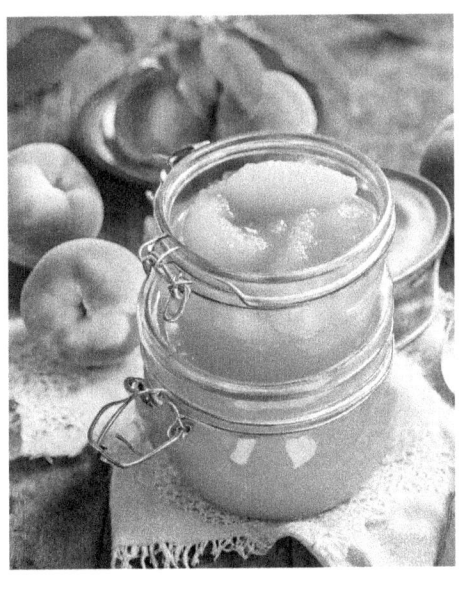

17. Baked Custard Oatmeal

Ingredients:
- 2 cups rolled oats
- 2 cups milk
- 2 large eggs
- 1/4 cup maple syrup or honey
- 1 teaspoon vanilla extract
- 1/2 teaspoon cinnamon
- 1/4 teaspoon salt

Instructions:
1. Preheat the oven to 350°F (175°C).
2. In a large bowl, whisk together milk, eggs, maple syrup, vanilla, cinnamon, and salt.
3. Stir in the oats and mix well.
4. Pour the mixture into a greased baking dish and bake for 35-40 minutes or until set and golden brown.
5. Let cool slightly before serving.

Servings: 6

Nutritional Information (per serving):
- Calories: 220
- Protein: 8g
- Carbohydrates: 36g
- Fat: 5g
- Fiber: 4g
- Sugar: 12g

Cooking Time: 45-50 minutes

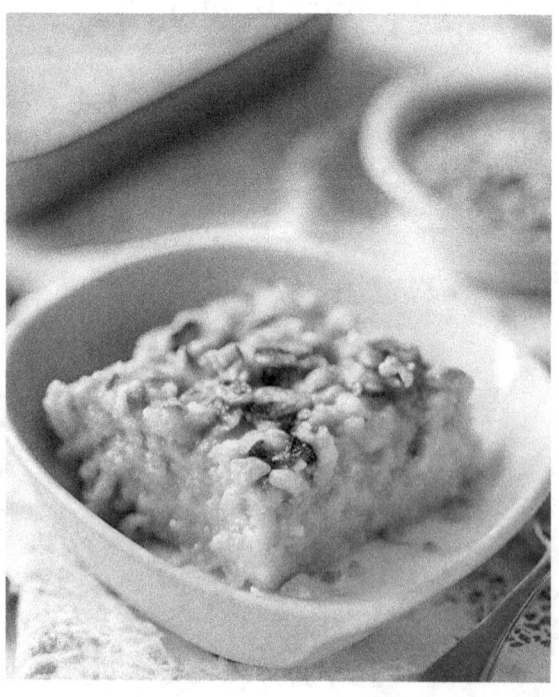

18. Chia Seed Pudding

Ingredients:
- 1/4 cup chia seeds
- 1 cup almond milk (or any milk of choice)
- 1 tablespoon maple syrup or honey
- 1/2 teaspoon vanilla extract

Instructions:
1. In a bowl, mix together chia seeds, almond milk, maple syrup, and vanilla.
2. Cover and refrigerate for at least 2 hours or overnight, until the mixture has thickened and become pudding-like.
3. 3. Stir the pudding before serving. If it's too thick, you can add a little more milk to reach your desired consistency.
4. Serve chilled, topped with fresh fruit or nuts if desired.

Servings: 2

Nutritional Information (per serving):
- Calories: 200
- Protein: 4g
- Carbohydrates: 24g
- Fat: 10g
- Fiber: 10g
- Sugar: 8g

Cooking Time: 2 hours (mostly refrigeration time)

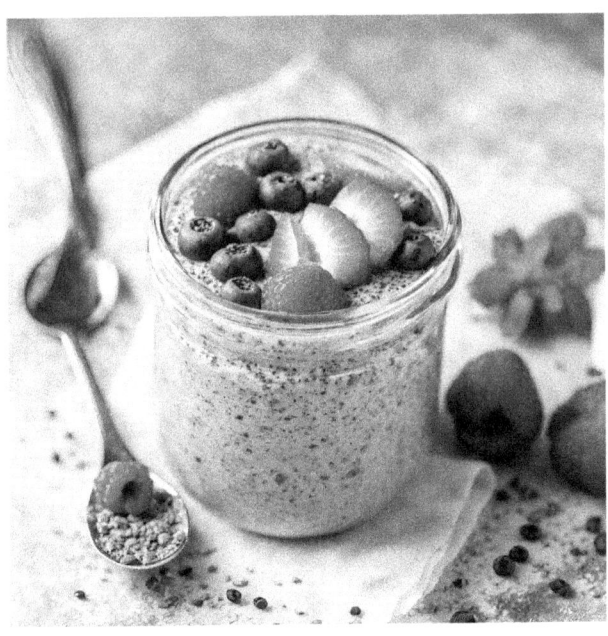

19. Rice Cakes with Avocado

Ingredients:
- 4 rice cakes
- 1 ripe avocado
- Salt and pepper to taste
- Lemon juice (optional)
- Toppings of choice: sliced cucumber, cherry tomatoes, radishes (optional)

Instructions:
1. Mash the avocado in a bowl and season with salt, pepper, and a squeeze of lemon juice if using.
2. Spread the mashed avocado evenly over the rice cakes.
3. Add additional toppings of your choice, such as sliced cucumber, cherry tomatoes, or radishes.
4. Serve immediately to maintain the crispiness of the rice cakes.

Servings: 2 (2 rice cakes each)

Nutritional Information (per serving):
- Calories: 240 (without additional toppings)
- Protein: 3g
- Carbohydrates: 30g
- Fat: 14g
- Fiber: 7g
- Sugar: 1g

Cooking Time: 10 minutes

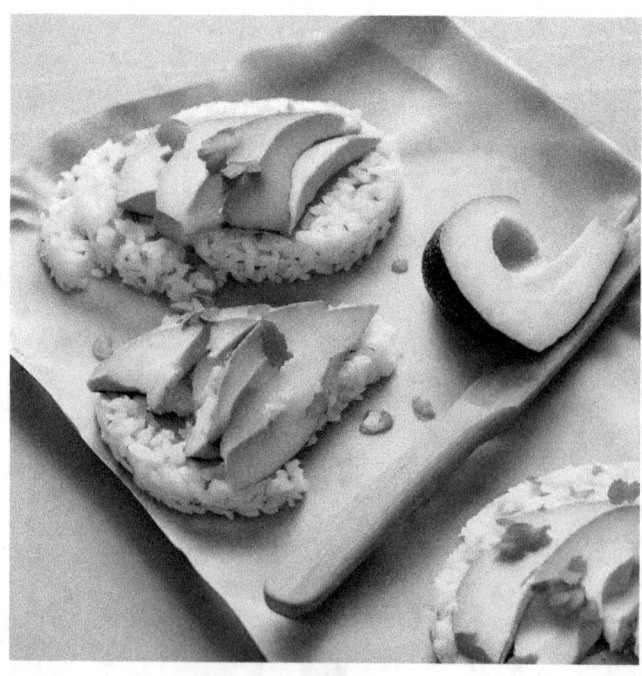

20. Silken Tofu Smoothie

Ingredients:
- 1 cup silken tofu
- 1 banana
- 1 cup fresh or frozen berries
- 1 cup almond milk or other plant-based milk
- 1 tablespoon honey or maple syrup (optional)
- Ice cubes (optional)

Instructions:
1. Combine the silken tofu, banana, berries, almond milk, and honey/maple syrup in a blender.
2. Add ice cubes if you prefer a colder smoothie.
3. Blend until smooth and creamy.
4. Taste and adjust sweetness if necessary, then blend again briefly.

Servings: 2

Nutritional Information (per serving):
- Calories: 200
- Protein: 9g
- Carbohydrates: 30g
- Fat: 5g
- Fiber: 4g
- Sugar: 16g (varies depending on the berries and sweetener used)

Cooking Time: 5 minutes

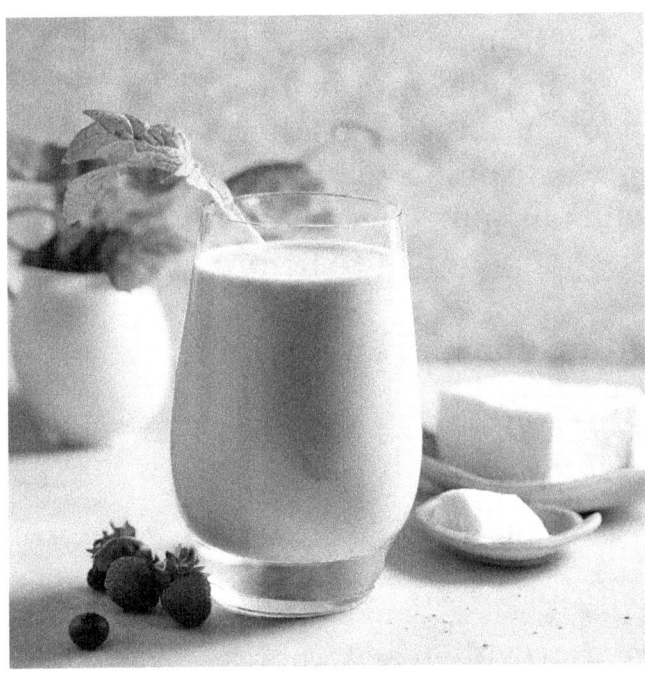

Poultry & Meat Recipes

1. Lamb Tagine
Ingredients:
- 2 lbs lamb shoulder, cut into chunks
- 2 tablespoons olive oil
- 1 large onion, finely chopped
- 2 cloves garlic, minced
- 2 teaspoons ground cumin
- 2 teaspoons ground coriander
- 1 teaspoon ground cinnamon
- 1/2 teaspoon ground ginger
- 1/2 teaspoon turmeric
- 2 cups beef or chicken broth
- 1 can (14 oz) diced tomatoes
- 1/2 cup dried apricots, chopped
- Salt and pepper to taste
- Fresh cilantro, chopped (for garnish)

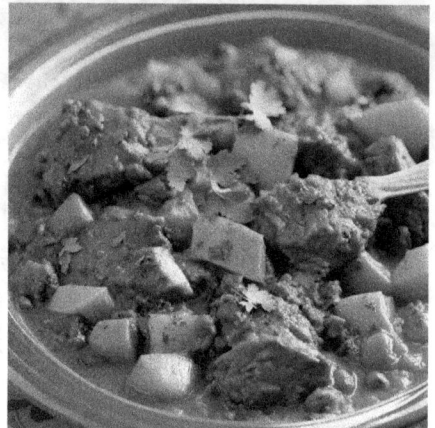

Instructions:
1. Heat olive oil in a large pot or Dutch oven over medium-high heat. Season the lamb with salt and pepper and brown in batches. Set aside.
2. In the same pot, add the onion and garlic, cooking until soft.
3. Return the lamb to the pot, and stir in the cumin, coriander, cinnamon, ginger, and turmeric until the lamb is well-coated.
4. Add the broth and diced tomatoes. Bring to a simmer, cover, and cook on low heat for 1.5 to 2 hours, until the lamb is tender.
5. Add the apricots and cook for another 30 minutes. Adjust seasoning with salt and pepper.
6. Garnish with chopped cilantro before serving.

Servings: 6
Nutritional Information (per serving):
- Calories: ~400
- Protein: ~35g
- Carbohydrates: ~20g
- Fat: ~20g
- Fiber: ~3g
- Sugar: ~10g

Cooking Time: Approximately 2.5 hours

2. Pork Chop Puree

Ingredients:
- 4 boneless pork chops
- 1 cup vegetable broth
- 1 tablespoon olive oil
- Salt and pepper to taste
- 1/2 cup heavy cream (optional for extra smoothness)

Instructions:
1. Season the pork chops with salt and pepper.
2. Heat olive oil in a skillet over medium-high heat and brown the pork chops on both sides.
3. Add the vegetable broth, cover, and simmer until the pork is very tender, about 25-30 minutes.
4. Remove the pork chops and let them cool slightly.
5. Blend the pork chops in a food processor or blender, adding cooking liquid as needed to achieve a smooth puree. For extra creaminess, add heavy cream during blending.
6. Adjust the seasoning and serve warm.

Servings: 4

Nutritional Information (per serving):
- Calories: ~250 (without heavy cream)
- Protein: ~29g
- Carbohydrates: ~1g
- Fat: ~14g (more with heavy cream)
- Fiber: 0g
- Sugar: 0g

Cooking Time: 35-40 minutes

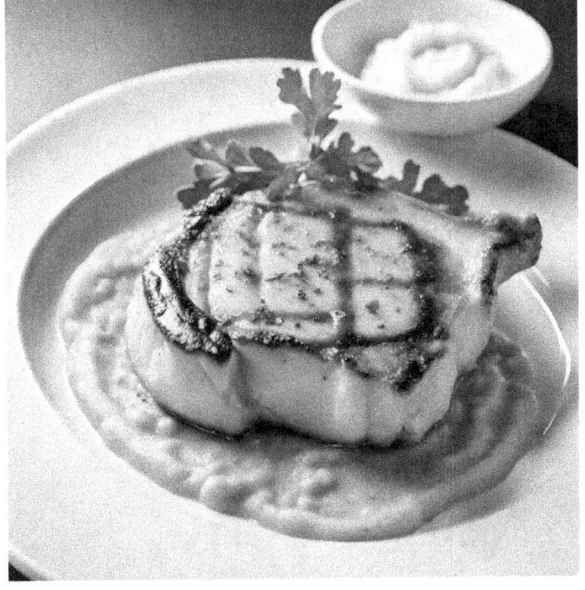

3. Chicken Tagine

Ingredients:
- 2 lbs chicken thighs, bone-in, skinless
- 2 tablespoons olive oil
- 1 large onion, chopped
- 2 garlic cloves, minced
- 1 teaspoon ground ginger
- 1 teaspoon ground turmeric
- 1/2 teaspoon ground cinnamon
- 1/2 teaspoon paprika
- 2 cups chicken broth
- 1 can (14 oz) chickpeas, drained and rinsed
- 1 cup dried apricots, halved
- Salt and pepper to taste
- Fresh parsley, chopped (for garnish)

Instructions:
1. Heat the olive oil in a large pot or Dutch oven over medium-high heat. Season the chicken with salt and pepper and brown on both sides. Remove and set aside.
2. In the same pot, add the onion and garlic, sautéing until softened.
3. Add the ginger, turmeric, cinnamon, and paprika, stirring for about 1 minute.
4. Return the chicken to the pot, add the chicken broth, chickpeas, and apricots. Bring to a simmer.
5. Cover and cook on low heat for about 1 hour, until the chicken is tender.
6. Season with salt and pepper, garnish with parsley, and serve.

Servings: 6

Nutritional Information (per serving):
- Calories: ~400
- Protein: ~35g
- Carbohydrates: ~30g
- Fat: ~15g
- Fiber: ~5g
- Sugar: ~15g

Cooking Time: 1.5 hours

4. Bison Meatballs

Ingredients:
- 1 lb ground bison
- 1/4 cup breadcrumbs
- 1 large egg
- 2 tablespoons milk
- 1/2 teaspoon garlic powder
- 1/2 teaspoon onion powder
- Salt and pepper to taste
- 2 tablespoons olive oil
- 2 cups tomato sauce (low sodium, if preferred)

Instructions:
1. In a large bowl, combine ground bison, breadcrumbs, egg, milk, garlic powder, onion powder, salt, and pepper. Mix until just combined.
2. Form the mixture into 1-inch meatballs.
3. Heat olive oil in a large skillet over medium heat. Add meatballs and brown on all sides, about 5-7 minutes.
4. Pour the tomato sauce over the meatballs, cover, and simmer on low heat for 20-25 minutes, or until meatballs are cooked through.
5. Serve hot, garnished with parsley or basil if desired.

Servings: 4

Nutritional Information (per serving):
- Calories: ~300 Protein: ~26g Carbohydrates: ~12g Fat: ~16g
- Fiber: ~2g
- Sugar: ~6g

Cooking Time: 35-40 minutes

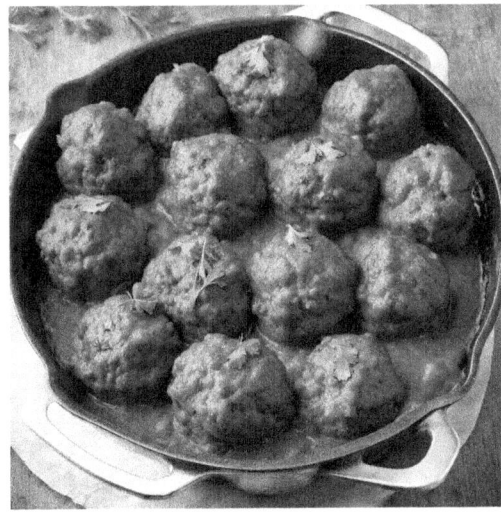

5. Grouper Fillets

Ingredients:
- 4 grouper fillets (6 ounces each)
- 2 tablespoons olive oil
- Salt and pepper to taste
- Lemon slices, for serving
- Fresh herbs (such as parsley or dill), for garnish

Instructions:
1. Preheat the oven to 375°F (190°C).
2. Brush both sides of the grouper fillets with olive oil and season with salt and pepper.
3. Place the fillets in a baking dish and bake for 10-12 minutes, or until the fish flakes easily with a fork.
4. Serve immediately with lemon slices and garnished with fresh herbs.

Servings: 4

Nutritional Information (per serving):
- Calories: ~240
- Protein: ~48g
- Carbohydrates: 0g
- Fat: ~5g
- Fiber: 0g
- Sugar: 0g

Cooking Time: 15-20 minutes

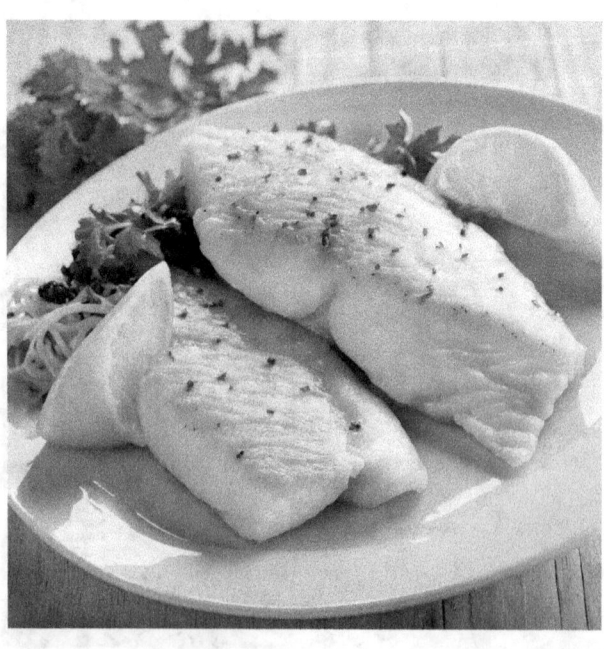

6. Veal Paprikash

Ingredients:
- 2 lbs veal, cut into 1-inch cubes
- 2 tablespoons olive oil
- 2 onions, finely chopped
- 2 garlic cloves, minced
- 2 tablespoons sweet paprika
- 1 cup beef broth
- 1 cup sour cream
- Salt and pepper to taste
- 1 tablespoon fresh parsley, chopped (for garnish)

Instructions:
1. Heat the olive oil in a large pot over medium-high heat. Add the veal cubes, season with salt and pepper, and brown them on all sides. Remove the veal and set aside.
2. In the same pot, add the onions and garlic, cooking until they are soft.
3. Stir in the paprika and cook for another minute.
4. Add the beef broth and return the veal to the pot. Bring to a simmer, then cover and cook on low heat for about 1 hour, until the veal is tender.
5. Stir in the sour cream and heat through (do not boil). Adjust seasoning with salt and pepper.
6. Garnish with parsley and serve with noodles or rice, if desired.

Servings: 6

Nutritional Information (per serving):
- Calories: ~350
- Protein: ~35g
- Carbohydrates: ~7g
- Fat: ~20g
- Fiber: ~1g
- Sugar: ~3g

Cooking Time: 1 hour 20 minutes

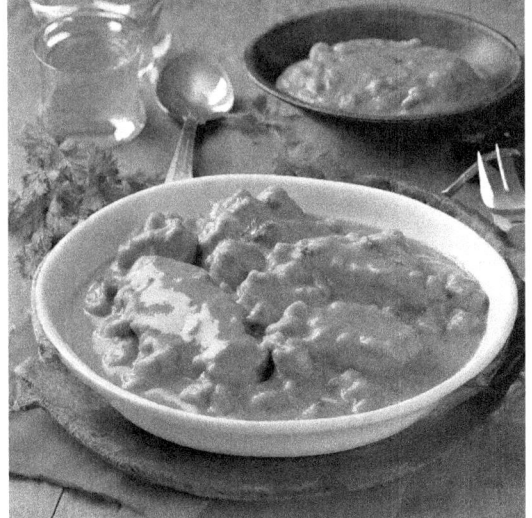

7. Beef Tenderloin

Ingredients:
- 2 lbs beef tenderloin
- 2 tablespoons olive oil
- Salt and pepper to taste
- 2 cloves garlic, minced
- 1 sprig rosemary (optional)

Instructions:
1. Preheat your oven to 400°F (200°C).
2. Rub the beef tenderloin with olive oil, then season generously with salt, pepper, and minced garlic.
3. If desired, place a sprig of rosemary on top.
4. Roast in the preheated oven until the meat reaches your desired doneness (about 20-25 minutes for medium-rare).
5. Let the meat rest for 10 minutes before slicing.

Servings: 6

Nutritional Information (per serving):
- Calories: ~450
- Protein: ~45g
- Carbohydrates: 0g
- Fat: ~30g
- Fiber: 0g
- Sugar: 0g

Cooking Time: 30-35 minutes (including resting time)

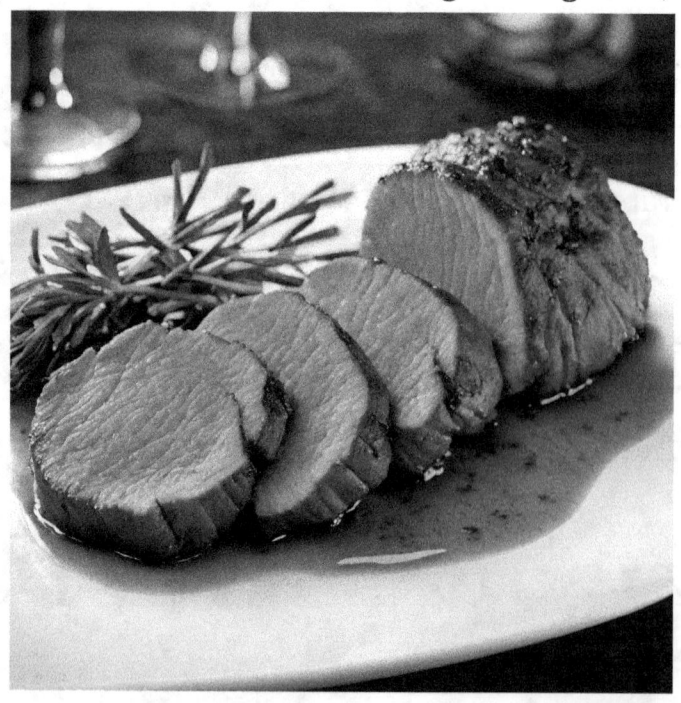

8. Pheasant Stew

Ingredients:
- 2 pheasants, cut into pieces
- 3 tablespoons olive oil
- 1 large onion, chopped
- 2 carrots, peeled and sliced
- 2 celery stalks, sliced
- 3 garlic cloves, minced
- 4 cups chicken broth
- 1 cup white wine (optional)
- Herbs (thyme, bay leaf)
- Salt and pepper to taste

Instructions:
1. In a large pot, heat olive oil over medium heat. Brown the pheasant pieces on all sides, then remove and set aside.
2. In the same pot, add the onion, carrots, celery, and garlic. Sauté until softened.
3. Deglaze the pot with white wine if using, then add the chicken broth and herbs.
4. Return the pheasant to the pot, cover, and simmer for about 1-1.5 hours until the pheasant is tender.
5. Season with salt and pepper to taste and serve.

Servings: 6

Nutritional Information (per serving):
- Calories: ~300
- Protein: ~35g
- Carbohydrates: ~8g
- Fat: ~10g
- Fiber: ~2g
- Sugar: ~3g

Cooking Time: 1.5-2 hours

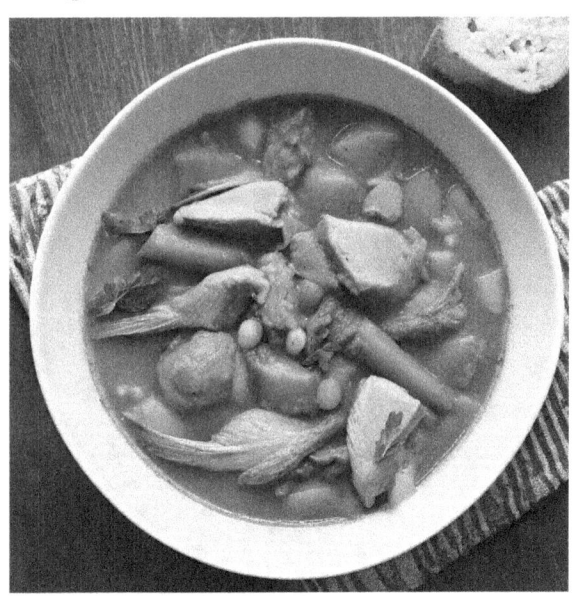

9. Roast Turkey Breast

Ingredients:
- 1 bone-in turkey breast (about 3-4 lbs)
- 2 tablespoons olive oil
- 1 tablespoon chopped fresh herbs (thyme, rosemary, sage)
- Salt and pepper to taste
- 2 cloves garlic, minced

Instructions:
1. Preheat your oven to 350°F (175°C).
2. Rub the turkey breast with olive oil and season with salt, pepper, minced garlic, and herbs.
3. Place in a roasting pan and roast until the internal temperature reaches 165°F (74°C), about 90 minutes.
4. Let rest for 10 minutes before slicing.

Servings: 6

Nutritional Information (per serving):
- Calories: ~320
- Protein: ~60g
- Carbohydrates: 0g
- Fat: ~7g
- Fiber: 0g
- Sugar: 0g

Cooking Time: About 1 hour 40 minutes (including resting time)

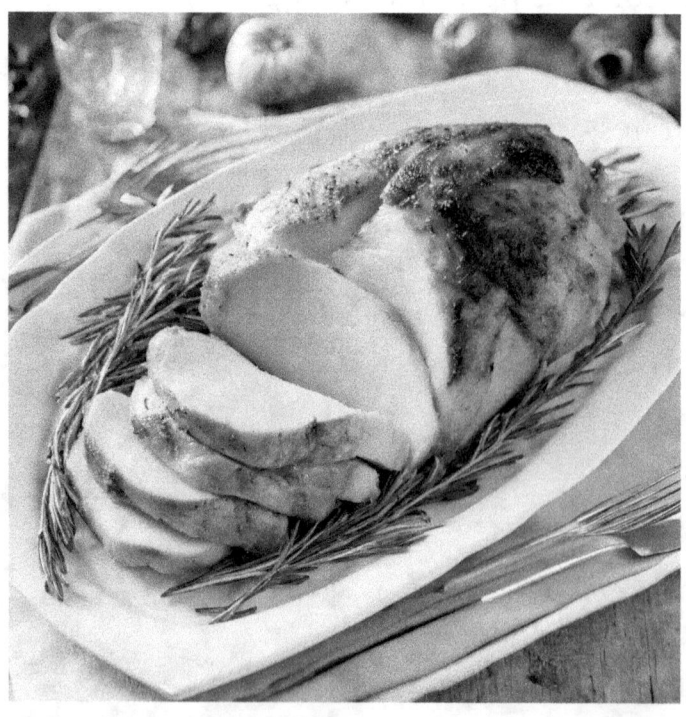

10. Chicken Porridge

Ingredients:
- 1 cup rice
- 6 cups chicken broth
- 1 lb boneless chicken breast, cut into small pieces
- 1 inch ginger, finely chopped
- Salt to taste

Instructions:
1. Rinse the rice until the water runs clear.
2. In a large pot, combine the rice, chicken broth, chicken, and ginger. Bring to a boil.
3. Reduce the heat to low, cover, and simmer for about 1 hour, stirring occasionally, until the mixture has a porridge-like consistency.
4. Season with salt to taste and serve warm.

Servings: 4-6

Nutritional Information (per serving for 6):
- Calories: ~220
- Protein: ~20g
- Carbohydrates: ~28g
- Fat: ~2g
- Fiber: ~0.5g
- Sugar: ~0.5g

Cooking Time: About 1 hour 10 minutes

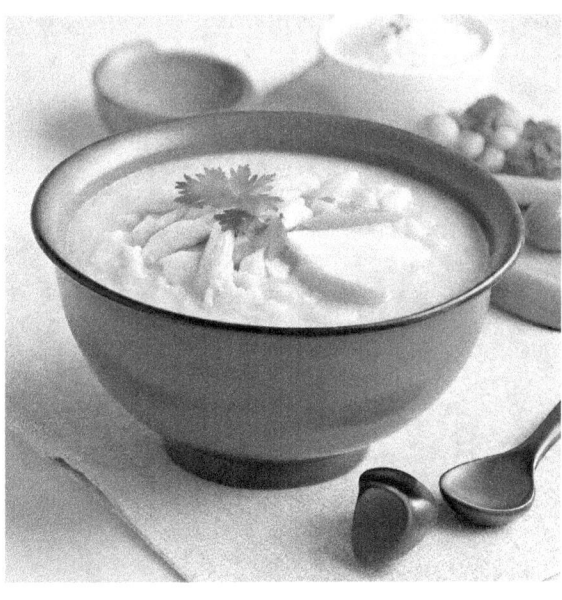

11. Duck Confit

Ingredients:
- 4 duck legs
- 4 cups duck fat (or enough to cover the duck legs)
- Salt and pepper to taste
- 4 garlic cloves, smashed
- 4 sprigs of thyme

Instructions:
1. Season the duck legs generously with salt and pepper. Place them in a dish, cover with plastic wrap, and refrigerate for at least 2 hours, preferably overnight.
2. Preheat your oven to 275°F (135°C).
3. Rinse the salt off the duck legs and pat them dry. Place them in a single layer in a deep baking dish. Add the garlic cloves and thyme, then pour the duck fat over the legs, ensuring they are completely submerged.
4. Cover the dish with foil and cook in the preheated oven for 2 to 3 hours, or until the meat is very tender and pulls away from the bone easily.
5. Let the duck cool in the fat, then you can store it in the fat until ready to use, or heat it under a broiler to crisp up the skin before serving.

Servings: 4

Nutritional Information (per serving):
- Calories: ~1300 (varies greatly depending on fat absorbed)
- Protein: ~31g   Carbohydrates: 0g
- Fat: ~120g (estimated; actual may vary)   Fiber: 0g   Sugar: 0g

Cooking Time: 2-3 hours (plus marinating time)

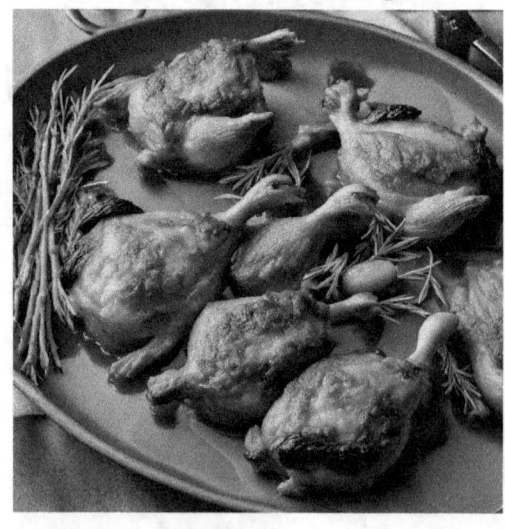

12. Braised Rabbit

Ingredients:
- 1 whole rabbit, cut into pieces
- 2 tablespoons olive oil
- 1 onion, chopped
- 2 carrots, diced
- 2 celery stalks, diced
- 4 garlic cloves, minced
- 1 cup white wine
- 2 cups chicken broth
- Herbs (rosemary, thyme)
- Salt and pepper to taste

Instructions:
1. Season the rabbit pieces with salt and pepper.
2. Heat olive oil in a large heavy pot over medium-high heat. Brown the rabbit pieces on all sides, then remove and set aside.
3. In the same pot, add the onion, carrots, celery, and garlic. Cook until softened.
4. Deglaze the pot with white wine, scraping up any browned bits.
5. Return the rabbit to the pot, add chicken broth, and herbs. Bring to a simmer.
6. Cover and cook on low heat for about 1.5 hours or until the rabbit is tender.
7. Season with additional salt and pepper to taste and serve.

Servings: 4-6

Nutritional Information (per serving for 6):
- Calories: ~300
- Protein: ~38g
- Carbohydrates: ~8g
- Fat: ~8g
- Fiber: ~1g
- Sugar: ~3g

Cooking Time: About 2 hours

13. Chicken Risotto

Ingredients:
- 1 lb chicken breast, diced
- 1 cup Arborio rice
- 4 cups chicken broth, warmed
- 1 onion, finely chopped
- 2 cloves garlic, minced
- 1/2 cup white wine (optional)
- 2 tablespoons olive oil
- 1/2 cup grated Parmesan cheese
- Salt and pepper to taste
- Fresh parsley, chopped (for garnish)

Instructions:
1. Heat 1 tablespoon olive oil in a large skillet over medium-high heat. Add chicken, season with salt and pepper, and cook until browned and cooked through. Set aside.
2. In the same skillet, add the remaining olive oil and sauté the onion and garlic until soft.
3. Add the Arborio rice, stirring to coat with the oil. Cook for 1-2 minutes.
4. If using, pour in the wine and let it evaporate.
5. Gradually add the warm chicken broth, one ladle at a time, stirring frequently, allowing each ladleful to be absorbed before adding the next, until the rice is al dente and creamy, about 18-20 minutes.
6. Stir in the cooked chicken and Parmesan cheese. Adjust the seasoning with salt and pepper.
7. Serve garnished with fresh parsley.

Servings: 4

Nutritional Information (per serving):
- Calories: ~500
- Protein: ~33g
- Carbohydrates: ~54g
- Fat: ~15g
- Fiber: ~1g
- Sugar: ~2g

Cooking Time: 30-35 minutes

14. Soft-Cooked Chicken Thighs

Ingredients:
- 4 chicken thighs, bone-in, skin-on
- 2 tablespoons olive oil
- Salt and pepper to taste
- 1 cup chicken broth
- 1 onion, finely chopped
- 2 cloves garlic, minced
- 1 teaspoon thyme (optional)

Instructions:
1. Preheat your oven to 375°F (190°C).
2. Season the chicken thighs with salt and pepper on both sides.
3. Heat olive oil in a large oven-proof skillet over medium-high heat. Add the chicken, skin-side down, and cook until the skin is golden and crisp, about 5-7 minutes. Flip the chicken and cook for another 3 minutes.
4. Remove the chicken and set aside. In the same skillet, add the onion and garlic, cooking until softened, about 2-3 minutes.
5. Return the chicken to the skillet, skin-side up, and add the chicken broth. Sprinkle with thyme if using.
6. Transfer the skillet to the oven and bake until the chicken is completely cooked through, reaching an internal temperature of 165°F (74°C), about 25-30 minutes.
7. Let the chicken rest for a few minutes before serving.

Servings: 4

Nutritional Information (per serving):
- Calories: ~350
- Protein: ~25g
- Carbohydrates: ~3g
- Fat: ~26g
- Fiber: ~0.5g
- Sugar: ~1g

Cooking Time: 40-45 minutes

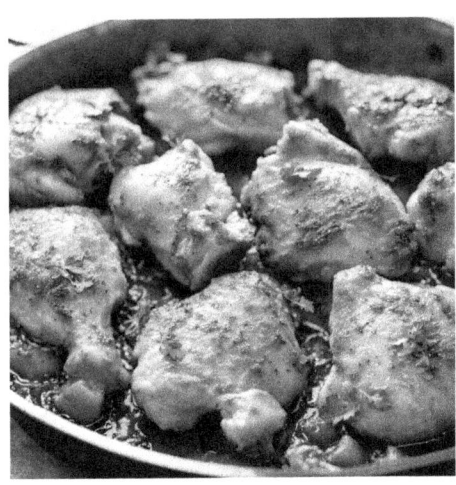

15. Veal Scallopini

Ingredients:
- 1 lb veal cutlets, pounded thin
- 1/4 cup all-purpose flour
- Salt and pepper to taste
- 4 tablespoons unsalted butter
- 1/2 cup white wine or chicken broth
- Juice of 1 lemon
- 2 tablespoons capers, rinsed (optional)
- 2 tablespoons chopped parsley (for garnish)

Instructions:
1. Season the veal cutlets with salt and pepper, then dredge them lightly in flour, shaking off any excess.
2. In a large skillet, melt 2 tablespoons of butter over medium-high heat. Add the veal cutlets and cook for about 2 minutes per side, or until they are golden brown and cooked through. Remove the veal from the skillet and set aside.
3. Add the white wine or chicken broth to the skillet, scraping up any browned bits from the bottom of the pan. Let it simmer and reduce by half, about 3-4 minutes.
4. Stir in the lemon juice, capers (if using), and remaining 2 tablespoons of butter. Cook for another minute until the sauce has thickened slightly.
5. Return the veal to the skillet, coating it in the sauce, and heat through for about 1 minute.
6. Serve the veal scallopini with the sauce poured over the top and garnished with chopped parsley.

Servings: 4

Nutritional Information (per serving):
- Calories: ~300
- Protein: ~24g
- Carbohydrates: ~5g
- Fat: ~18g
- Fiber: ~0.1g
- Sugar: ~0.2g

Cooking Time: 20 minutes

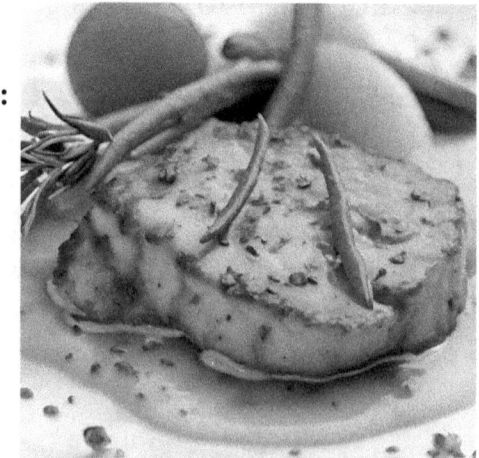

16. Lamb Puree

Ingredients:
- 1 lb lamb stew meat
- 2 cups beef broth
- Salt and pepper to taste
- 1 bay leaf (optional)
- 1/4 cup cooked carrots (optional for sweetness)

Instructions:
1. Place the lamb, beef broth, salt, pepper, and bay leaf in a saucepan.
2. Bring to a boil, then reduce heat to low, cover, and simmer until the lamb is very tender, about 2 hours.
3. Remove the bay leaf and transfer the lamb and a bit of the cooking liquid (and cooked carrots if using) to a blender.
4. Puree until smooth, adding more cooking liquid as needed to reach desired consistency.
5. Season with additional salt and pepper to taste.

Servings: 4

Nutritional Information (per serving):
- Calories: ~300
- Protein: ~24g
- Carbohydrates: ~0g (without carrots)
- Fat: ~22g
- Fiber: 0g

Cooking Time: About 2 hours

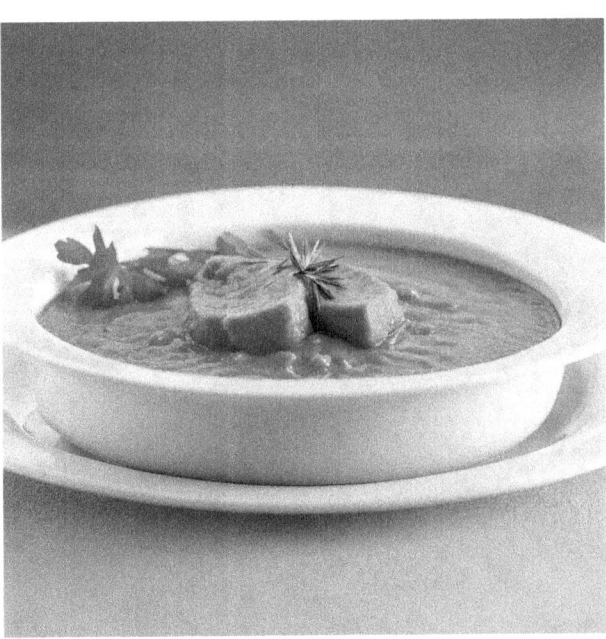

17. Turkey Patties

Ingredients:
- 1 lb ground turkey
- 1/4 cup breadcrumbs
- 1 egg, beaten
- 1 tablespoon olive oil
- Salt and pepper to taste
- 1/2 teaspoon garlic powder (optional)
- 1/2 teaspoon onion powder (optional)

Instructions:
1. Combine the ground turkey, breadcrumbs, beaten egg, salt, pepper, garlic powder, and onion powder in a bowl. Mix well.
2. Form the mixture into small patties.
3. Heat olive oil in a skillet over medium heat and cook the patties for about 5 minutes per side or until fully cooked.
4. Serve hot.

Servings: 4

Nutritional Information (per serving):
- Calories: ~240
- Protein: ~27g
- Carbohydrates: ~6g
- Fat: ~12g
- Fiber: ~0.5g

Cooking Time: 20 minutes

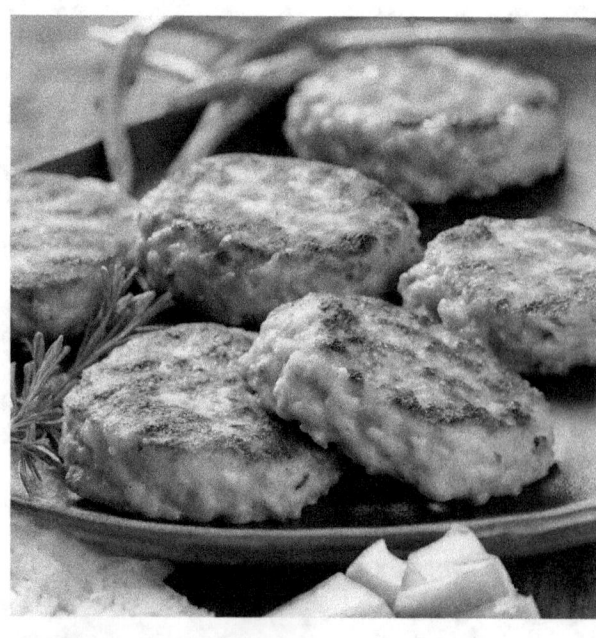

18. Oven-Poached Salmon

Ingredients:
- 4 salmon fillets (6 oz each)
- 1 cup white wine or water
- Lemon slices
- Fresh dill or parsley
- Salt and pepper to taste

Instructions:
1. Preheat the oven to 350°F (175°C).
2. Season the salmon fillets with salt and pepper and place them in a baking dish.
3. Pour the white wine or water into the dish and add lemon slices and herbs around the salmon.
4. Cover the dish with foil and bake for 15-20 minutes, or until the salmon flakes easily with a fork.
5. Serve garnished with additional fresh herbs.

Servings: 4

Nutritional Information (per serving):
- Calories: ~350
- Protein: ~34g
- Carbohydrates: ~0g
- Fat: ~20g
- Fiber: 0g

Cooking Time: 25-30 minutes

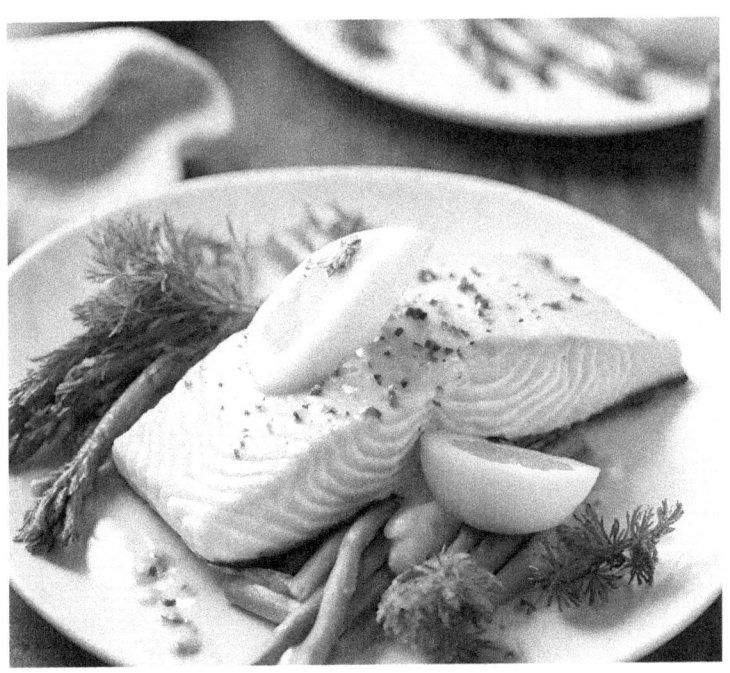

19. Beef Stew

Ingredients:
- 2 lbs beef stew meat, cubed
- 4 cups beef broth
- 2 carrots, peeled and sliced (optional)
- 2 potatoes, peeled and cubed (optional)
- 1 onion, chopped (optional)
- Salt and pepper to taste
- 2 tablespoons olive oil
- 2 tablespoons tomato paste (optional)
- 1 teaspoon thyme

Instructions:
1. Heat olive oil in a large pot over medium-high heat. Brown the beef cubes on all sides, then remove from the pot.
2. (Optional) In the same pot, add the onion, carrots, and potatoes and sauté until softened.
3. Return the beef to the pot, add the beef broth, tomato paste, thyme, salt, and pepper.
4. Bring to a boil, then reduce heat to low, cover, and simmer for about 1.5-2 hours, until the beef is tender.
5. Adjust the seasoning and serve hot.

Servings: 6

Nutritional Information (per serving):
- Calories: ~400 Protein: ~35g
- Carbohydrates: ~15g (without vegetables)
- Fat: ~20g
- Fiber: ~2g

Cooking Time: 2-2.5 hours

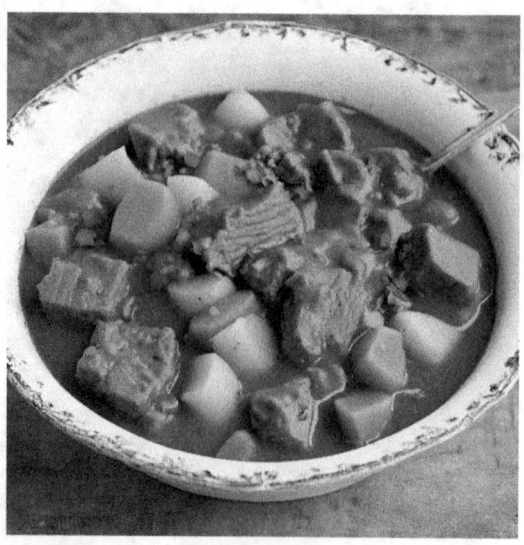

20. Pulled Pork

Ingredients:
- 3 lbs pork shoulder
- 1 cup barbecue sauce (choose a low-sugar variety for a healthier option)
- 1/2 cup apple cider vinegar
- 1/2 cup chicken broth
- 2 tablespoons light brown sugar (optional)
- 1 tablespoon mustard
- 1 tablespoon Worcestershire sauce
- 1 teaspoon paprika
- Salt and pepper to taste

Instructions:
1. Season the pork shoulder with salt and pepper, and place it in a slow cooker.
2. In a bowl, combine the barbecue sauce, apple cider vinegar, chicken broth, brown sugar (if using), mustard, Worcestershire sauce, and paprika. Stir well to combine.
3. Pour the mixture over the pork in the slow cooker.
4. Cover and cook on low for 8-10 hours or on high for 4-5 hours, until the pork is very tender and shreds easily with a fork.
5. Remove the pork from the slow cooker and shred it using two forks. If desired, skim off any fat from the sauce remaining in the slow cooker and discard.
6. Return the shredded pork to the slow cooker and stir into the sauce. Allow it to soak up the flavors for an additional 30 minutes.
7. Serve the pulled pork warm, either on its own or as a filling for sandwiches.

Servings: 8

Nutritional Information (per serving):
- Calories: ~380
- Protein: ~35g
- Carbohydrates: ~15g (adjust for sugar and barbecue sauce used)
- Fat: ~20g
- Fiber: ~0g

Cooking Time: 8-10 hours on low, or 4-5 hours on high

21. Poached Chicken Breast

Ingredients:
- 4 boneless, skinless chicken breasts
- 4 cups chicken broth or water
- 1 onion, quartered (optional)
- 2 garlic cloves, crushed (optional)
- 2 bay leaves (optional)
- Salt and pepper to taste

Instructions:
1. In a large pot, add the chicken breasts. Cover them with the chicken broth or water. Add the onion, garlic, bay leaves, salt, and pepper if using.
2. Bring the mixture to a boil, then immediately reduce the heat to low, ensuring the liquid is at a gentle simmer.
3. Poach the chicken for about 15-20 minutes, or until the internal temperature reaches 165°F (74°C) and the meat is no longer pink inside.
4. Remove the chicken from the pot and let it rest for a few minutes before slicing or shredding.
5. The poached chicken can be served as is, or used in salads, sandwiches, or other dishes.

Servings: 4

Nutritional Information (per serving):
- Calories: ~160
- Protein: ~31g
- Carbohydrates: ~0g (unless vegetables are eaten)
- Fat: ~3g
- Fiber: 0g

Cooking Time: 25-30 minutes

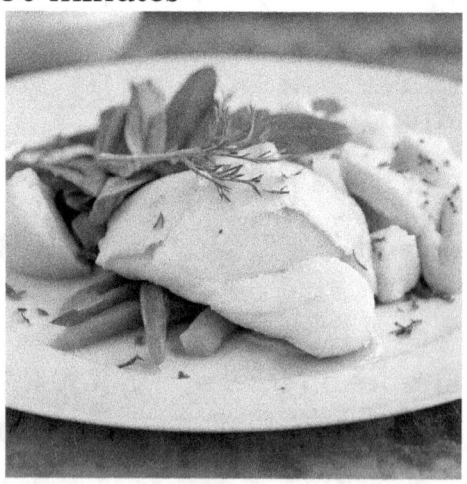

VEGETABLES

1. Fennel Puree
Ingredients:
- 2 large fennel bulbs, chopped
- 2 tablespoons olive oil
- 1/2 cup vegetable broth
- Salt and pepper to taste
- 1/4 cup heavy cream (optional)

Instructions:
1. In a large saucepan, heat the olive oil over medium heat. Add the chopped fennel and sauté until tender, about 10-15 minutes.
2. Add the vegetable broth, cover, and simmer until the fennel is very soft, about 15-20 minutes.
3. Remove from heat and let cool slightly. Transfer to a blender, adding the heavy cream if using, and puree until smooth.
4. Season with salt and pepper to taste. Serve warm.

Servings: 4

Nutritional Information (per serving):
- Calories: ~120 (without cream) Protein: ~2g
- Carbohydrates: ~10g
- Fat: ~8g
- Fiber: ~4g

Cooking Time: 35-40 minutes

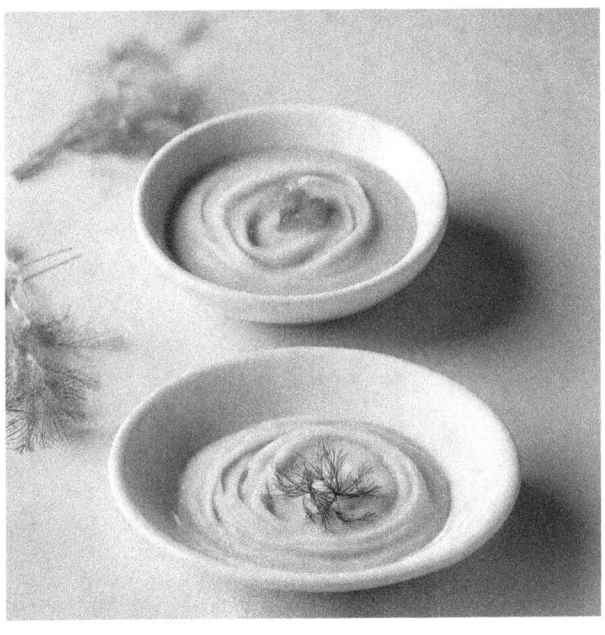

2. Bamboo Shoots

Ingredients:
- 1 can (14 oz) bamboo shoots, drained
- 1 tablespoon sesame oil
- 1 tablespoon soy sauce
- 1 teaspoon sugar (optional)
- 1 garlic clove, minced (optional)

Instructions:
1. Rinse the bamboo shoots under cold water and drain.
2. Heat the sesame oil in a skillet over medium heat. Add the minced garlic if using, and sauté until fragrant.
3. Add the bamboo shoots and stir-fry for 5-7 minutes.
4. Add the soy sauce and sugar, stirring well to coat the bamboo shoots. Cook for an additional 2-3 minutes.
5. Serve warm as a side dish.

Servings: 4

Nutritional Information (per serving):
- Calories: ~60
- Protein: ~2g
- Carbohydrates: ~4g
- Fat: ~4g
- Fiber: ~1g

Cooking Time: 10-15 minutes

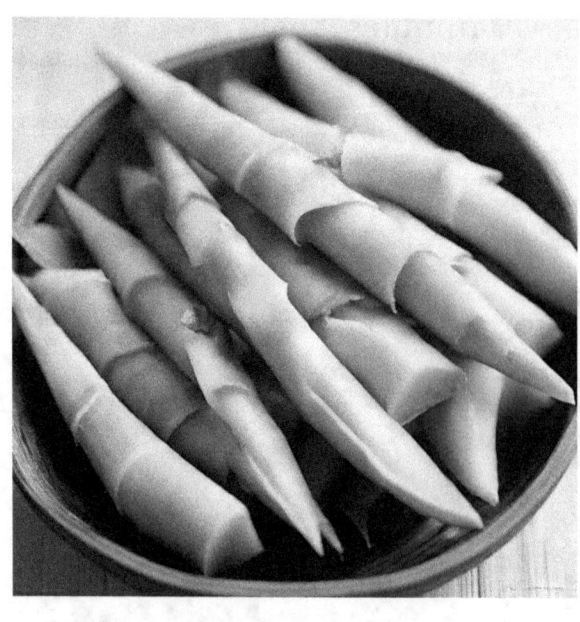

3. Watercress Soup

Ingredients:
- 2 bunches watercress, roughly chopped
- 1 tablespoon olive oil
- 1 onion, chopped
- 2 potatoes, peeled and diced
- 4 cups vegetable broth
- Salt and pepper to taste
- 1/2 cup heavy cream (optional)

Instructions:
1. In a large pot, heat the olive oil over medium heat. Add the onion and sauté until translucent.
2. Add the potatoes and vegetable broth. Bring to a boil, then reduce heat and simmer until the potatoes are tender, about 15 minutes.
3. Add the watercress and cook for an additional 3-5 minutes, until wilted but still bright green.
4. Remove from heat and let cool slightly. Puree the soup in batches in a blender until smooth.
5. Return the soup to the pot, stir in the heavy cream if using, and reheat gently. Season with salt and pepper to taste.
6. Serve hot.

Servings: 4

Nutritional Information (per serving):
- Calories: ~150 (without cream)
- Protein: ~3g
- Carbohydrates: ~18g
- Fat: ~7g
- Fiber: ~3g

Cooking Time: 30 minutes

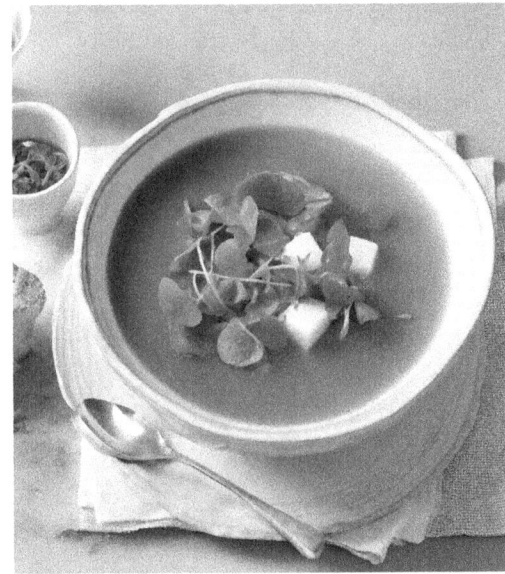

4. Stewed Tomatoes

Ingredients:
- 4 large tomatoes, chopped
- 1 tablespoon olive oil
- 1 onion, finely chopped
- 2 cloves garlic, minced
- Salt and pepper to taste
- 1 teaspoon dried basil or oregano (optional)

Instructions:
1. Heat the olive oil in a saucepan over medium heat. Add the onion and garlic, and sauté until softened.
2. Add the chopped tomatoes and herbs if using. Season with salt and pepper.
3. Cover and simmer on low heat for 15-20 minutes, stirring occasionally, until the tomatoes are soft and the flavors have melded.
4. Serve warm as a side dish or over cooked grains.

Servings: 4

Nutritional Information (per serving):
- Calories: ~80
- Protein: ~2g
- Carbohydrates: ~10g
- Fat: ~4g
- Fiber: ~2g

Cooking Time: 25-30 minutes

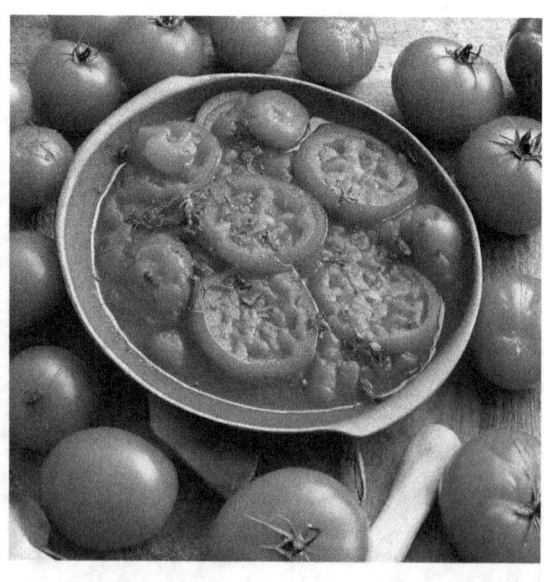

5. Mushroom Broth

Ingredients:
- 1 lb fresh mushrooms, chopped
- 1 onion, chopped
- 2 cloves garlic, minced
- 6 cups water
- 2 tablespoons olive oil
- Salt and pepper to taste
- A few sprigs of thyme or parsley (optional)

Instructions:
1. In a large pot, heat the olive oil over medium heat. Add the onion and garlic, and sauté until translucent.
2. Add the mushrooms and cook, stirring occasionally, until they release their juices and begin to brown, about 10 minutes.
3. Add the water and bring the mixture to a boil. Reduce the heat to low, add the thyme or parsley if using, and simmer uncovered for about 1 hour.
4. Strain the broth through a fine-mesh sieve, discarding the solids. Season the broth with salt and pepper to taste.
5. Serve hot or use as a base for soups and sauces.

Servings: 6

Nutritional Information (per serving):
- Calories: ~70
- Protein: ~3g
- Carbohydrates: ~6g
- Fat: ~4g
- Fiber: ~1g

Cooking Time: About 1 hour 15 minutes

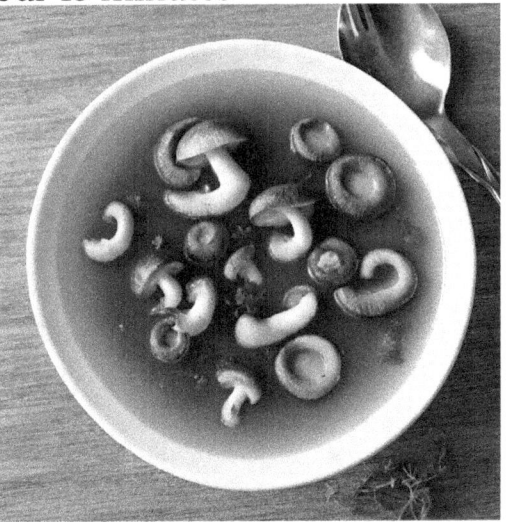

6. Turnip Soup

Ingredients:
- 3 large turnips, peeled and diced
- 1 tablespoon olive oil
- 1 onion, chopped
- 2 cloves garlic, minced
- 4 cups vegetable broth
- Salt and pepper to taste
- 1/2 cup heavy cream (optional)

Instructions:
1. In a large pot, heat the olive oil over medium heat. Add the onion and garlic, and sauté until soft.
2. Add the diced turnips and cook for a few minutes until they start to become tender.
3. Pour in the vegetable broth, season with salt and pepper, and bring to a boil. Reduce heat and simmer for about 20 minutes or until the turnips are very soft.
4. Remove from heat and let cool slightly. Puree the soup in batches in a blender until smooth.
5. Return the soup to the pot and stir in the heavy cream if using. Heat gently, adjust the seasoning, and serve.

Servings: 4

Nutritional Information (per serving):
- Calories: ~120 (without cream)
- Protein: ~2g
- Carbohydrates: ~12g
- Fat: ~7g
- Fiber: ~3g

Cooking Time: 30-40 minutes

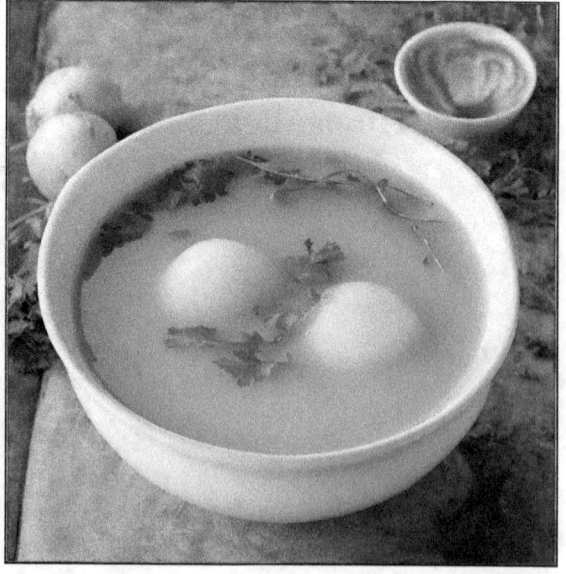

7. Celery Root Puree

Ingredients:
- 2 large celery roots (celeriac), peeled and cubed
- 3 tablespoons unsalted butter
- 1/2 cup milk or cream
- Salt and white pepper to taste

Instructions:
1. Place the cubed celery root in a large pot and cover with water. Bring to a boil, then reduce heat and simmer until tender, about 20-30 minutes.
2. Drain the celery root and return it to the pot. Add butter and milk or cream.
3. Mash the mixture with a potato masher or puree it with an immersion blender until smooth. Season with salt and white pepper to taste.
4. Serve warm as a side dish, similar to mashed potatoes.

Servings: 4

Nutritional Information (per serving):
- Calories: ~180
- Protein: ~2g
- Carbohydrates: ~18g
- Fat: ~12g
- Fiber: ~3g

Cooking Time: 35-40 minutes

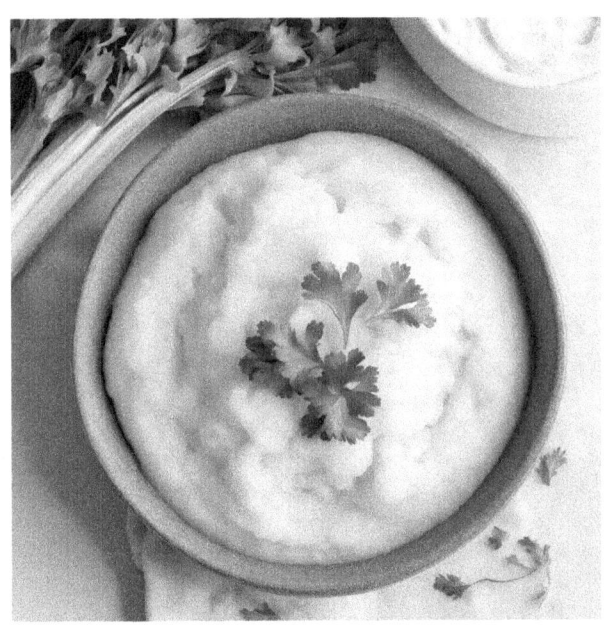

8. Jicama Slaw

Ingredients:
- 1 large jicama, peeled and julienned
- 1 carrot, peeled and julienned (optional)
- 1/4 cup lime juice
- 2 tablespoons olive oil
- 1 tablespoon honey or agave syrup
- Salt and pepper to taste
- 2 tablespoons chopped cilantro or parsley

Instructions:
1. In a large bowl, combine the julienned jicama and carrot.
2. In a small bowl, whisk together the lime juice, olive oil, honey, salt, and pepper.
3. Pour the dressing over the jicama and carrots, tossing to coat evenly.
4. Chill in the refrigerator for at least 30 minutes to allow the flavors to meld.
5. Just before serving, toss with fresh cilantro or parsley.

Servings: 4

Nutritional Information (per serving):
- Calories: ~130
- Protein: ~1g
- Carbohydrates: ~20g
- Fat: ~5g
- Fiber: ~6g

Cooking Time: 10 minutes (plus chilling time)

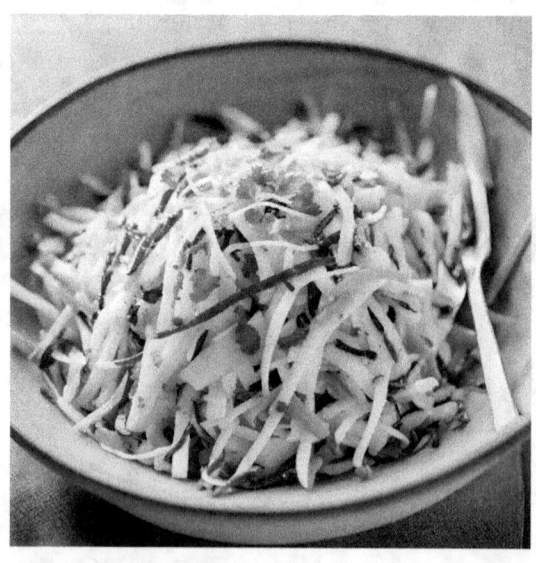

9. Kabocha Squash Soup

Ingredients:
- 1 medium kabocha squash, peeled, seeded, and cubed
- 1 tablespoon olive oil
- 1 onion, chopped
- 3 cups vegetable broth
- Salt and pepper to taste
- 1/2 cup coconut milk

Instructions:
1. Heat olive oil in a large pot over medium heat. Add the onion and sauté until translucent.
2. Add the kabocha squash and vegetable broth. Season with salt and pepper.
3. Bring to a boil, then reduce heat and simmer until the squash is tender, about 20-30 minutes.
4. Puree the soup using an immersion blender or in batches in a regular blender until smooth.
5. Stir in the coconut milk and heat through. Adjust seasoning if necessary.
6. Serve hot.

Servings: 4

Nutritional Information (per serving):
- Calories: ~150
- Protein: ~2g
- Carbohydrates: ~20g
- Fat: ~7g
- Fiber: ~5g

Cooking Time: 40-45 minutes

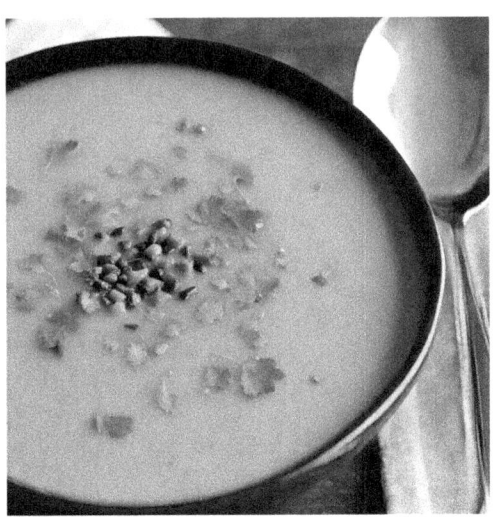

10. Plantain Porridge

Ingredients:
- 2 ripe plantains, peeled and chopped
- 4 cups milk (or a non-dairy alternative)
- 1 cinnamon stick
- Sugar or honey to taste (optional)
- A pinch of salt

Instructions:
1. Combine the plantains, milk, cinnamon stick, and a pinch of salt in a saucepan.
2. Bring to a low boil, then reduce heat and simmer gently until the plantains are very soft, about 25-30 minutes.
3. Remove the cinnamon stick. Blend the mixture using an immersion blender or regular blender until smooth.
4. Return the porridge to the pot. Add sugar or honey to taste, if desired. Heat through.
5. Serve warm, garnished with a sprinkle of cinnamon if liked.

Servings: 4

Nutritional Information (per serving):
- Calories: ~250 (varies with sweetener)
- Protein: ~5g
- Carbohydrates: ~50g
- Fat: ~3.5g (more with full-fat milk)
- Fiber: ~3g

Cooking Time: 35-40 minutes

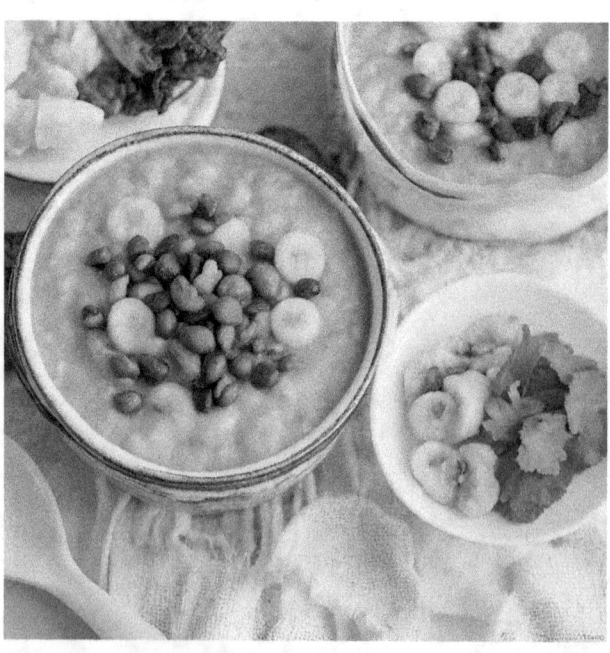

11. Chayote Mash

Ingredients:
- 2 large chayotes, peeled, seeded, and chopped
- 2 tablespoons butter or olive oil
- Salt and pepper to taste
- 1/4 cup milk or cream (optional)

Instructions:
1. Boil the chayote pieces in salted water until very tender, about 15-20 minutes.
2. Drain the chayotes and return them to the pot.
3. Add the butter or olive oil, and mash the chayotes until they reach your desired consistency.
4. Stir in milk or cream if using, and season with salt and pepper.
5. Serve warm.

Servings: 4

Nutritional Information (per serving):
- Calories: ~100 (more with cream)
- Protein: ~1g
- Carbohydrates: ~9g
- Fat: ~7g (with butter)
- Fiber: ~4g

Cooking Time: 25-30 minutes

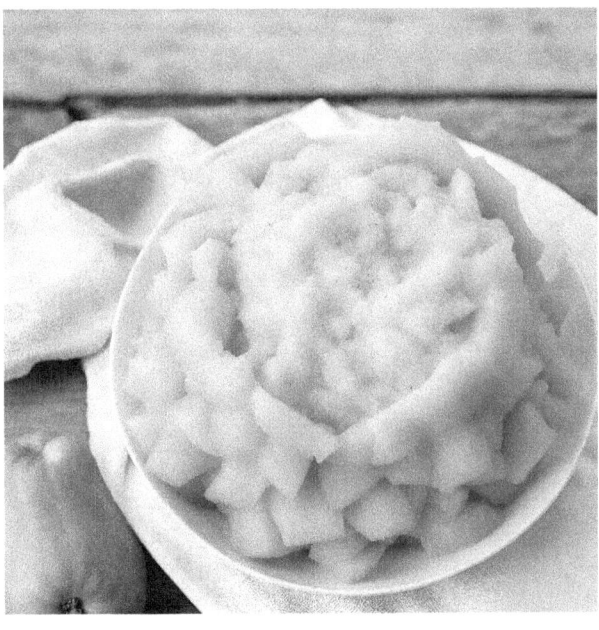

12. Okra Stew

Ingredients:
- 1 lb okra, trimmed and sliced
- 2 tablespoons olive oil
- 1 onion, diced
- 2 cloves garlic, minced
- 1 can (14 oz) diced tomatoes
- 2 cups vegetable broth
- Salt and pepper to taste
- 1 teaspoon paprika (optional)

Instructions:
1. Heat olive oil in a large pot over medium heat. Add the onion and garlic, and sauté until softened.
2. Add the okra, diced tomatoes, vegetable broth, salt, pepper, and paprika. Stir to combine.
3. Bring to a simmer and cook, covered, until the okra is tender, about 20-25 minutes.
4. Adjust the seasoning and serve hot.

Servings: 4

Nutritional Information (per serving):
- Calories: ~130
- Protein: ~3g
- Carbohydrates: ~15g
- Fat: ~7g
- Fiber: ~5g

Cooking Time: 35-40 minutes

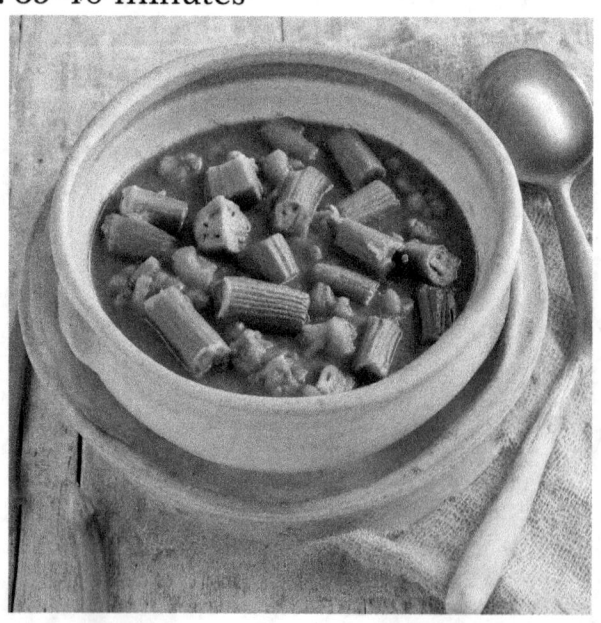

13. Sweet Corn Puree

Ingredients:
- 4 cups fresh sweet corn kernels (from about 4-5 ears of corn)
- 1 cup water or vegetable broth
- 2 tablespoons butter
- Salt to taste

Instructions:
1. Combine the corn and water/broth in a medium saucepan over medium heat.
2. Bring to a simmer and cook until the corn is tender, about 10-15 minutes.
3. Remove from heat and allow to cool slightly.
4. Transfer the corn mixture to a blender, add the butter, and puree until smooth. You may need to do this in batches depending on the size of your blender.
5. Return the puree to the saucepan and reheat gently. Season with salt to taste.
6. Serve warm as a side dish or a base for other recipes.

Servings: 4

Nutritional Information (per serving):
- Calories: ~190
- Protein: ~5g
- Carbohydrates: ~31g
- Fat: ~7g
- Fiber: ~4g

Cooking Time: 20-25 minutes

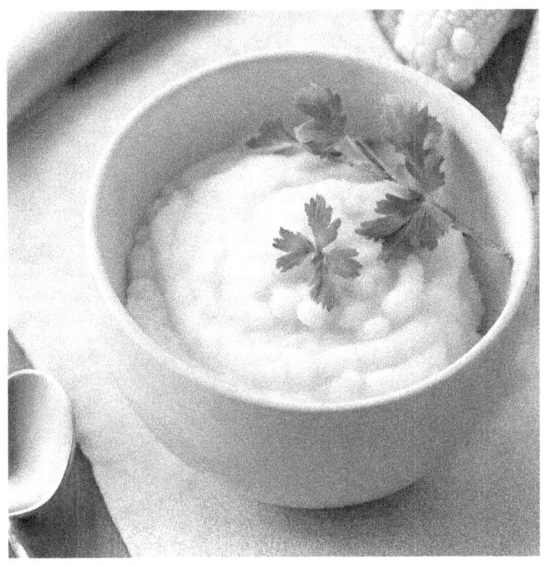

14. Daikon Radish Salad

Ingredients:
- 2 large daikon radishes, peeled and julienned
- 1 carrot, peeled and julienned (optional)
- 2 tablespoons rice vinegar
- 1 tablespoon sesame oil
- 1 teaspoon sugar or honey
- Salt to taste
- 1 tablespoon sesame seeds (optional)

Instructions:
1. In a large bowl, combine the julienned daikon and carrot.
2. In a small bowl, whisk together the rice vinegar, sesame oil, sugar or honey, and salt until well combined.
3. Pour the dressing over the daikon and carrot mixture and toss to coat evenly.
4. Let the salad sit for at least 15 minutes to marinate, tossing occasionally.
5. Sprinkle with sesame seeds before serving, if using.

Servings: 4

Nutritional Information (per serving):
- Calories: ~80
- Protein: ~1g
- Carbohydrates: ~10g
- Fat: ~4g
- Fiber: ~2g

Cooking Time: 20 minutes (including marinating time)

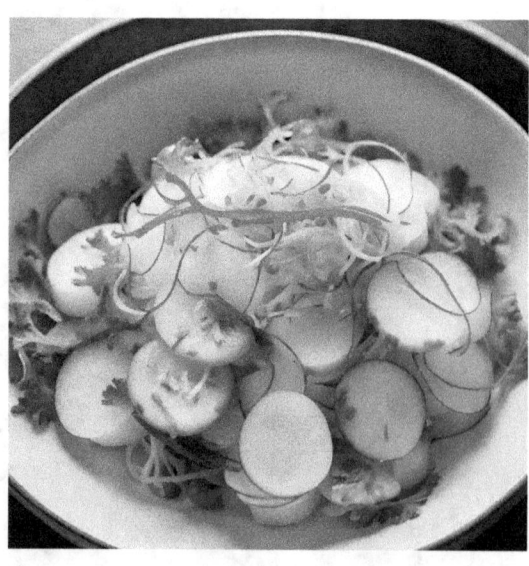

15. Roasted Parsnips

Ingredients:
- 1 lb parsnips, peeled and sliced into sticks
- 2 tablespoons olive oil
- Salt and pepper to taste
- Fresh herbs (like thyme or rosemary), finely chopped (optional)

Instructions:
1. Preheat the oven to 425°F (220°C).
2. Toss the parsnips with olive oil, salt, pepper, and herbs if using.
3. Spread the parsnips out in a single layer on a baking sheet.
4. Roast for 20-25 minutes, or until golden brown and tender, turning once halfway through.
5. Serve warm as a side dish.

Servings: 4

Nutritional Information (per serving):
- Calories: ~140
- Protein: ~1g
- Carbohydrates: ~20g
- Fat: ~7g
- Fiber: ~6g

Cooking Time: 30-35 minutes

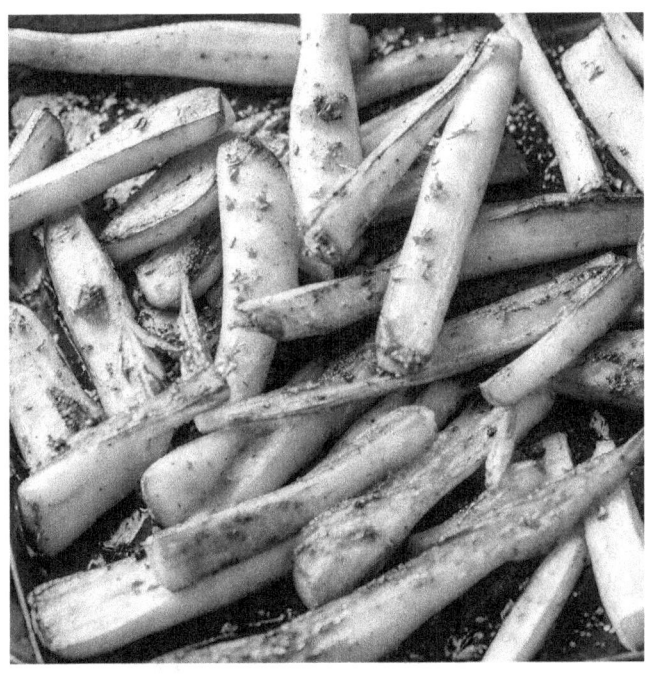

16. Asparagus Soup

Ingredients:
- 1 lb asparagus, trimmed and cut into 1-inch pieces
- 1 tablespoon olive oil
- 1 onion, chopped
- 2 cloves garlic, minced
- 3 cups vegetable broth
- Salt and pepper to taste
- 1/2 cup heavy cream or coconut milk (optional)

Instructions:
1. Heat olive oil in a large pot over medium heat. Add onion and garlic, and sauté until soft.
2. Add the asparagus and cook for an additional 5 minutes.
3. Pour in the vegetable broth, season with salt and pepper, and bring to a simmer. Cook until the asparagus is very tender, about 15-20 minutes.
4. Use an immersion blender to puree the soup until smooth, or transfer to a blender in batches and blend until smooth.
5. If desired, stir in the heavy cream or coconut milk and warm through. Adjust seasoning if needed.
6. Serve hot, garnished with asparagus tips or fresh herbs if desired.

Servings: 4

Nutritional Information (per serving):
- Calories: ~150 (with heavy cream)
- Protein: ~4g
- Carbohydrates: ~10g
- Fat: ~11g (with olive oil and heavy cream)
- Fiber: ~3g

Cooking Time: 30-35 minutes

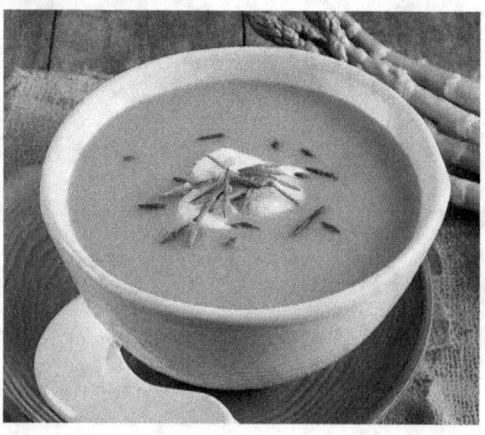

17. Silken Tofu and Bok Choy

Ingredients:
- 1 block silken tofu, drained
- 4 baby bok choy, cleaned and sliced in half lengthwise
- 2 tablespoons soy sauce
- 1 tablespoon sesame oil
- 1 teaspoon grated ginger
- 1 garlic clove, minced (optional, depending on tolerance)
- 1 tablespoon olive oil

Instructions:
1. Heat olive oil in a large skillet over medium heat. Add the bok choy and sauté until the leaves start to wilt and the stems are tender, about 5-7 minutes.
2. In a small bowl, mix soy sauce, sesame oil, grated ginger, and minced garlic.
3. Gently place the tofu in the skillet, being careful not to break it. Pour the soy sauce mixture over the tofu and bok choy.
4. Cover and let simmer gently for 3-5 minutes, allowing the tofu to warm through and absorb the flavors.
5. Serve warm, being careful to keep the tofu intact.

Servings: 4

Nutritional Information (per serving):
- Calories: ~150
- Protein: ~10g
- Carbohydrates: ~5g
- Fat: ~10g
- Fiber: ~1g

Cooking Time: 15 minutes

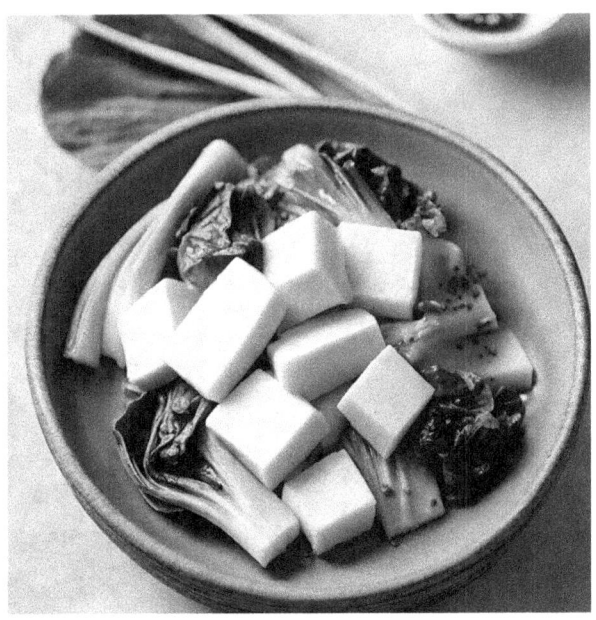

18. Beetroot Salad

Ingredients:
- 4 medium beetroots, cooked, peeled, and diced
- 2 tablespoons olive oil
- 1 tablespoon balsamic vinegar
- Salt and pepper to taste
- Fresh parsley, chopped (optional)

Instructions:
1. In a large bowl, combine the diced beetroots, olive oil, balsamic vinegar, salt, and pepper. Toss to coat evenly.
2. Refrigerate for at least 1 hour to allow flavors to meld.
3. Serve chilled, garnished with fresh parsley if desired.

Servings: 4

Nutritional Information (per serving):
- Calories: ~120
- Protein: ~2g
- Carbohydrates: ~13g
- Fat: ~7g
- Fiber: ~3g

Cooking Time: 1 hour 10 minutes (including chilling time)

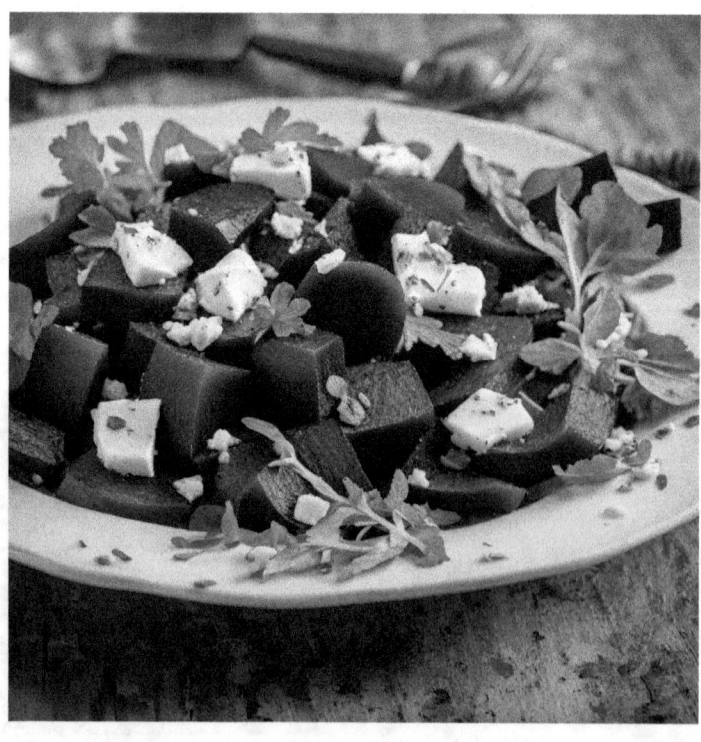

19. Eggplant Dip

Ingredients:
- 1 large eggplant
- 2 tablespoons olive oil
- 1 garlic clove, minced (optional)
- 1 tablespoon tahini
- Juice of 1 lemon
- Salt and pepper to taste

Instructions:
1. Preheat the oven to 400°F (200°C). Prick the eggplant with a fork and place it on a baking sheet.
2. Roast the eggplant until it's completely soft and the skin is charred, about 40-50 minutes.
3. Let the eggplant cool, then peel and discard the skin. Place the eggplant flesh in a blender.
4. Add olive oil, minced garlic (if using), tahini, lemon juice, salt, and pepper to the blender. Blend until smooth.
5. Adjust seasoning as needed and serve chilled or at room temperature.

Servings: 4

Nutritional Information (per serving):
- Calories: ~140
- Protein: ~2g
- Carbohydrates: ~10g
- Fat: ~10g
- Fiber: ~5g

Cooking Time: 50-60 minutes

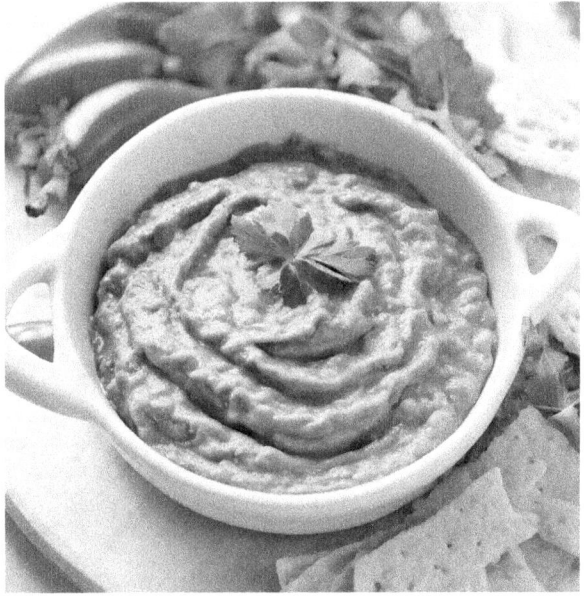

20. Pureed Peas

Ingredients:
- 2 cups frozen peas, thawed
- 2 tablespoons butter
- Salt and pepper to taste
- 1/4 cup cream or milk (optional)

Instructions:
1. In a medium saucepan, heat the peas, butter, and a splash of water over medium heat until the peas are heated through and tender, about 5-7 minutes.
2. Transfer the peas to a blender, add cream or milk if using, and puree until smooth.
3. Season with salt and pepper to taste, and serve warm.

Servings: 4

Nutritional Information (per serving):
- Calories: ~120 (with cream)
- Protein: ~4g
- Carbohydrates: ~12g
- Fat: ~6g
- Fiber: ~4g

Cooking Time: 10-15 minutes

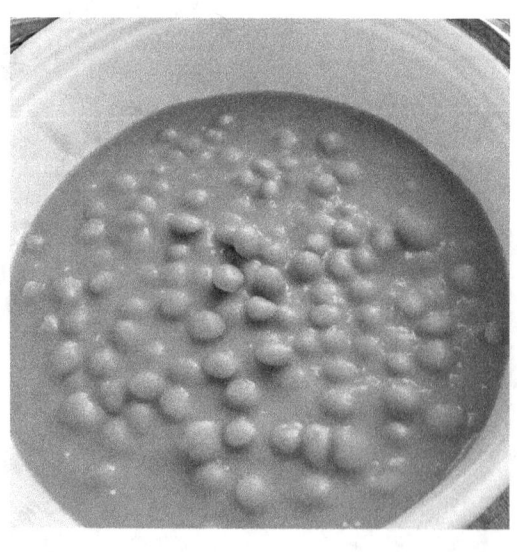

21. Zucchini Ribbons

Ingredients:
- 2 large zucchinis
- 2 tablespoons olive oil
- Salt and pepper to taste
- Lemon zest or juice (optional)

Instructions:
1. Use a vegetable peeler or mandoline slicer to slice the zucchinis into long, thin ribbons.
2. Heat the olive oil in a large skillet over medium heat. Add the zucchini ribbons, tossing gently to coat with the oil.
3. Sauté the ribbons for 2-3 minutes until they are just tender. Be careful not to overcook; they should retain a bit of their crispness.
4. Season with salt and pepper to taste, and add a touch of lemon zest or a squeeze of lemon juice if desired for extra flavor.
5. Serve immediately, either as a side dish or as a base for a light salad.

Servings: 4

Nutritional Information (per serving):
- Calories: ~90
- Protein: ~2g
- Carbohydrates: ~4g
- Fat: ~7g
- Fiber: ~1g

Cooking Time: 5-10 minutes

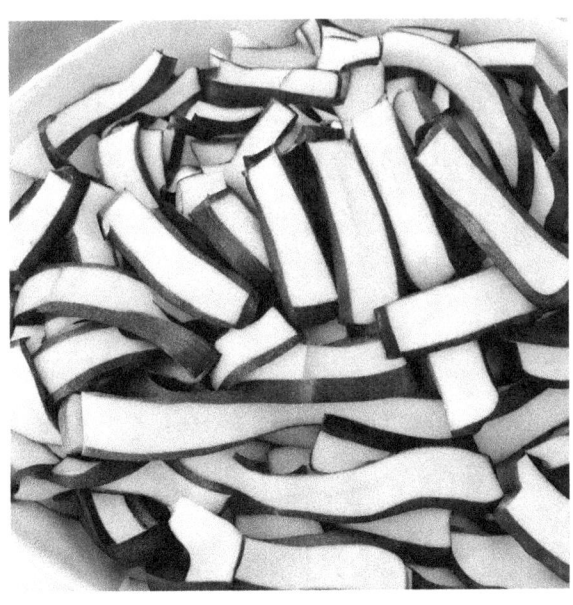

22. Carrot Soup

Ingredients:
- 1 lb carrots, peeled and chopped
- 1 tablespoon olive oil
- 1 onion, chopped
- 2 cloves garlic, minced (optional, if tolerated)
- 4 cups vegetable broth
- Salt and pepper to taste
- 1/2 cup coconut milk or cream (optional, for richness)

Instructions:
1. Heat the olive oil in a large pot over medium heat. Add the onions and sauté until translucent. Add the garlic if using and cook for another minute.
2. Add the chopped carrots to the pot along with the vegetable broth. Season with salt and pepper.
3. Bring to a boil, then reduce heat to low and simmer until the carrots are very tender, about 20-30 minutes.
4. Use an immersion blender to puree the soup directly in the pot, or carefully transfer to a blender in batches and puree until smooth.
5. If using, stir in the coconut milk or cream and warm through. Adjust the seasoning as needed.
6. Serve hot, garnished with a drizzle of cream or a sprinkle of fresh herbs if desired.

Servings: 4

Nutritional Information (per serving):
- Calories: ~120 (without coconut milk)
- Protein: ~2g
- Carbohydrates: ~15g
- Fat: ~6g (with olive oil)
- Fiber: ~4g

Cooking Time: 35-40 minutes

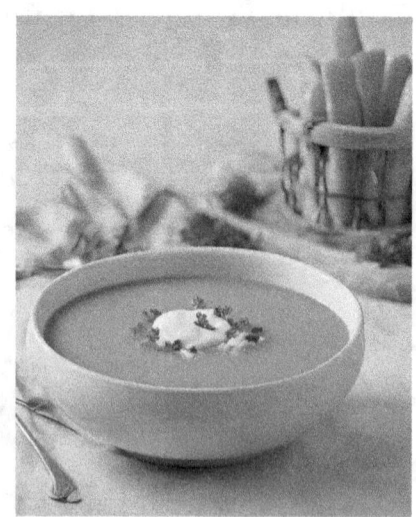

FISH AND SEAFOOD

1. Shrimp and Rice Congee
Ingredients:
- 1 cup jasmine rice
- 8 cups water or low-sodium chicken broth
- 1 lb shrimp, peeled and deveined
- 1-inch piece of ginger, peeled and minced
- Salt to taste
- 2 green onions, chopped
- Soy sauce and sesame oil for serving (optional)

Instructions:
1. Rinse the rice until the water runs clear, then combine it with the water or broth in a large pot.
2. Bring to a boil, then reduce heat to a low simmer. Cook, stirring occasionally, until the rice is broken down and the mixture has a porridge-like consistency, about 1.5 to 2 hours.
3. Add the shrimp and ginger to the congee during the last 10 minutes of cooking, ensuring the shrimp are cooked through.
4. Season with salt, and serve hot, garnished with green onions and a drizzle of soy sauce and sesame oil if desired.

Servings: 4-6
Nutritional Information (per serving, for 6 servings):
- Calories: ~220
- Protein: ~20g
- Carbohydrates: ~30g
- Fat: ~2g
- Fiber: ~1g

Cooking Time: About 2 hours

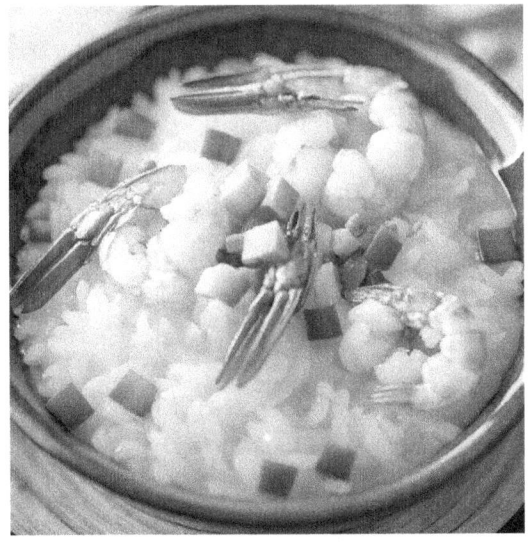

2. Lingcod in Pesto

Ingredients:
- 4 lingcod fillets (about 6 oz each)
- 4 tablespoons pesto sauce (store-bought or homemade)
- Salt and pepper to taste
- Lemon wedges for serving

Instructions:
1. Preheat the oven to 375°F (190°C).
2. Season the lingcod fillets with salt and pepper and spread each fillet with 1 tablespoon of pesto sauce.
3. Place the fillets in a baking dish and bake until the fish flakes easily with a fork, about 15-20 minutes.
4. Serve hot with lemon wedges on the side.

Servings: 4

Nutritional Information (per serving):
- Calories: ~300
- Protein: ~40g
- Carbohydrates: ~2g
- Fat: ~14g (varies with pesto used)
- Fiber: ~0.5g

Cooking Time: 20-25 minutes

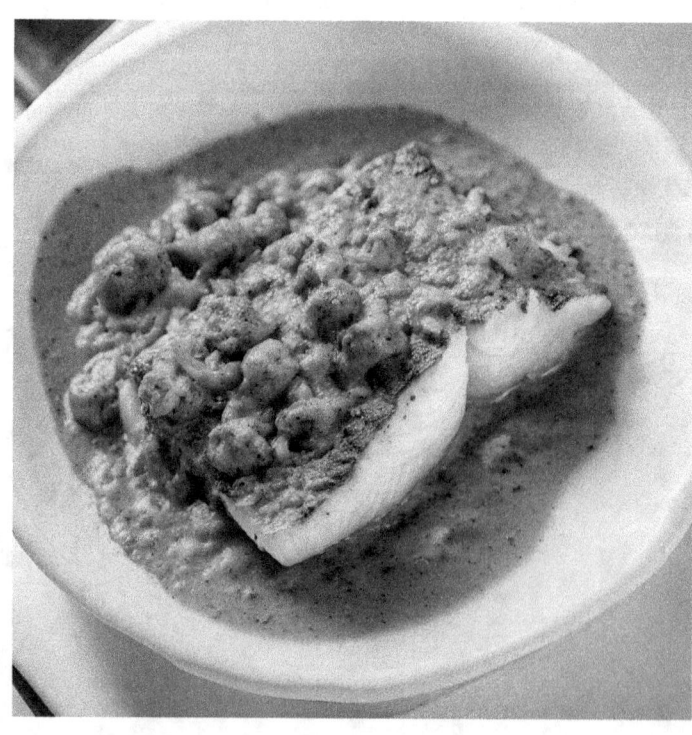

3. Monkfish Medallions

Ingredients:
- 1 lb monkfish tail, cut into 1-inch medallions
- 2 tablespoons olive oil
- Salt and pepper to taste
- 1/4 cup white wine
- 1 tablespoon lemon juice
- 1 tablespoon chopped parsley

Instructions:
1. Season the monkfish medallions with salt and pepper.
2. Heat the olive oil in a skillet over medium-high heat. Add the monkfish and cook until golden brown on both sides, about 3-4 minutes per side.
3. Add the white wine and lemon juice to the skillet, reduce the heat to low, and cover. Simmer until the fish is cooked through, about 5-7 minutes.
4. Garnish with chopped parsley and serve.

Servings: 4

Nutritional Information (per serving):
- Calories: ~200
- Protein: ~23g
- Carbohydrates: ~1g
- Fat: ~10g
- Fiber: 0g

Cooking Time: 15-20 minutes

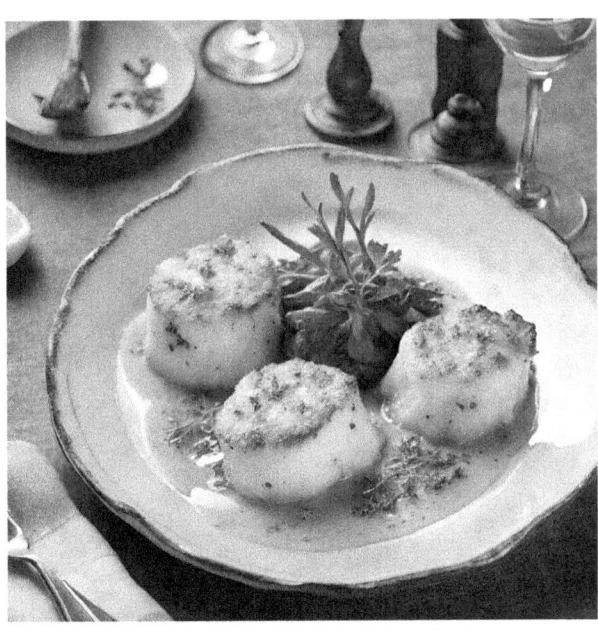

4. Squid Ink Pasta

Ingredients:
- 8 oz squid ink pasta
- 2 tablespoons olive oil
- 2 garlic cloves, minced
- 1/2 lb shrimp, peeled and deveined
- 1/2 lb calamari rings
- 1/2 cup white wine
- Salt and pepper to taste
- Chopped parsley for garnish

Instructions:
1. Cook the squid ink pasta according to package instructions until al dente. Drain and set aside.
2. In a large skillet, heat the olive oil over medium heat. Add the garlic and sauté until fragrant, about 1 minute.
3. Add the shrimp and calamari and cook until the shrimp turn pink and the calamari is tender, about 3-5 minutes.
4. Deglaze the pan with white wine and simmer for an additional 2 minutes. Season with salt and pepper.
5. Toss the cooked pasta with the seafood mixture. Garnish with parsley and serve.

Servings: 4

Nutritional Information (per serving):
- Calories: ~350
- Protein: ~25g
- Carbohydrates: ~45g
- Fat: ~7g
- Fiber: ~2g

Cooking Time: 20-30 minutes

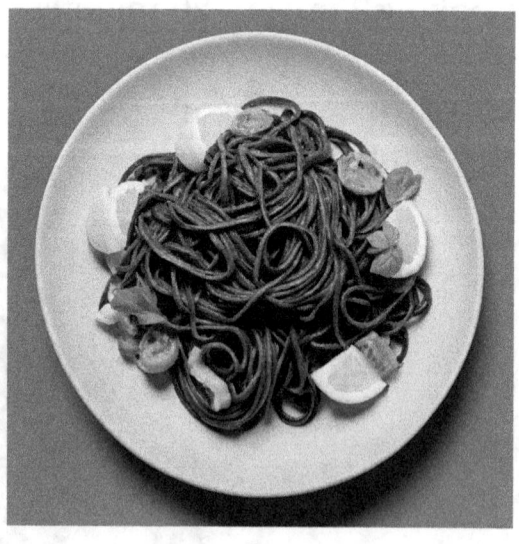

5. Bouillabaisse

Ingredients:
- 1 lb mixed seafood (such as shrimp, scallops, mussels, and firm white fish)
- 2 tablespoons olive oil
- 1 onion, chopped
- 2 cloves garlic, minced
- 1 fennel bulb, thinly sliced
- 1 can (14 oz) diced tomatoes
- 4 cups fish or vegetable broth
- 1 pinch saffron threads (optional)
- 1 teaspoon orange zest
- Salt and pepper to taste
- Fresh parsley, chopped for garnish

Instructions:
1. In a large pot, heat the olive oil over medium heat. Add the onion, garlic, and fennel, and sauté until softened, about 5-7 minutes.
2. Add the diced tomatoes, broth, saffron (if using), and orange zest. Season with salt and pepper. Bring to a simmer.
3. Add the mixed seafood to the pot, cover, and cook until the seafood is cooked through, about 5-10 minutes, depending on the size of the pieces.
4. Adjust the seasoning as needed. Ladle the soup into bowls and garnish with fresh parsley.

Servings: 4

Nutritional Information (per serving):
- Calories: ~300
- Protein: ~35g
- Carbohydrates: ~15g
- Fat: ~10g
- Fiber: ~3g

Cooking Time: 30-40 minutes

6. Sole Florentine

Ingredients:
- 4 sole fillets (about 6 oz each)
- 2 cups fresh spinach, steamed and chopped
- 2 tablespoons butter
- 2 tablespoons all-purpose flour
- 1 cup milk
- Salt and pepper to taste
- Nutmeg, a pinch
- 1/2 cup grated Parmesan cheese

Instructions:
1. Preheat the oven to 350°F (175°C).
2. Lay the sole fillets flat and divide the steamed spinach among them, placing it on one end of each fillet. Roll up the fillets and place them seam-side down in a baking dish.
3. In a saucepan, melt the butter over medium heat. Stir in the flour to make a roux, cooking for 1 minute. Gradually whisk in the milk until the sauce thickens. Season with salt, pepper, and a pinch of nutmeg.
4. Pour the sauce over the rolled fillets and sprinkle with Parmesan cheese.
5. Bake in the preheated oven until the fish is cooked through and the top is golden, about 20-25 minutes.

Servings: 4

Nutritional Information (per servin
- Calories: ~280
- Protein: ~28g
- Carbohydrates: ~8g
- Fat: ~15g
- Fiber: ~1g

Cooking Time: 35-45 minutes

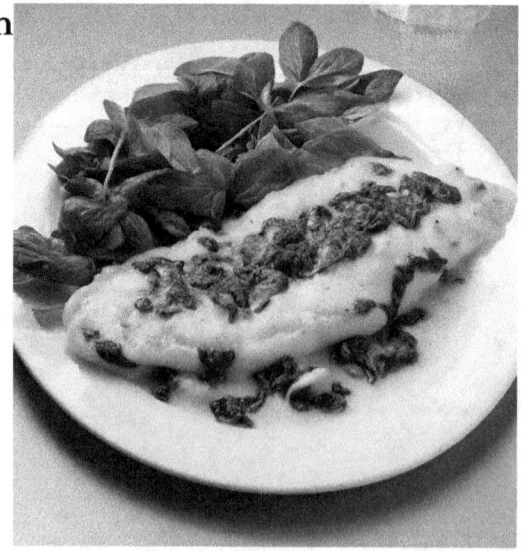

7. Snapper Veracruz

Ingredients:
- 4 snapper fillets (about 6 oz each)
- 2 tablespoons olive oil
- 1 onion, sliced
- 3 garlic cloves, minced
- 1 can (14 oz) diced tomatoes
- 1/4 cup green olives, sliced
- 2 tablespoons capers
- 1/2 teaspoon dried oregano
- Salt and pepper to taste
- 1/4 cup chopped fresh cilantro

Instructions:
1. Heat the olive oil in a large skillet over medium heat. Add the onion and garlic, and sauté until softened.
2. Stir in the diced tomatoes, olives, capers, and oregano. Season with salt and pepper. Cook for about 5 minutes to blend the flavors.
3. Place the snapper fillets in the sauce, spooning some over the top. Cover and simmer until the fish is cooked through, about 10-15 minutes.
4. Garnish with chopped cilantro and serve.

Servings: 4

Nutritional Information (per serving):
- Calories: ~300
- Protein: ~35g
- Carbohydrates: ~10g
- Fat: ~14g
- Fiber: ~2g

Cooking Time: 25-30 minutes

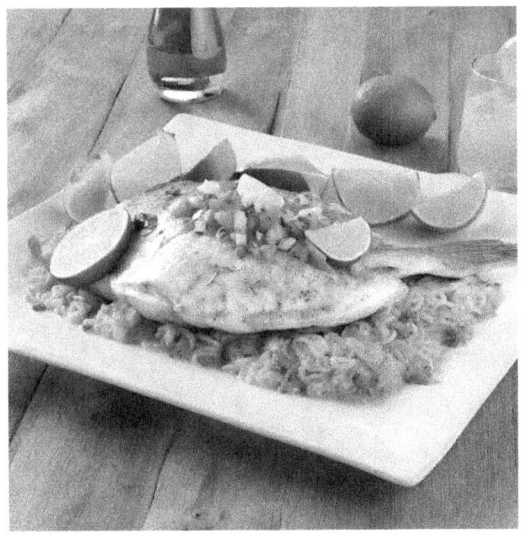

8. Barramundi with Lime

Ingredients:
- 4 barramundi fillets (about 6 oz each)
- 2 tablespoons olive oil
- Salt and pepper to taste
- 2 limes, one juiced and one cut into wedges
- Fresh herbs (such as cilantro or parsley), for garnish

Instructions:
1. Preheat the oven to 400°F (200°C).
2. Season the barramundi fillets with salt and pepper. Drizzle with olive oil and half of the lime juice.
3. Place the fillets in a baking dish, and bake until the fish flakes easily with a fork and is opaque throughout, about 12-15 minutes.
4. Remove from the oven and drizzle with the remaining lime juice.
5. Serve immediately, garnished with fresh herbs and accompanied by lime wedges.

Servings: 4

Nutritional Information (per serving):
- Calories: ~230
- Protein: ~23g
- Carbohydrates: ~1g
- Fat: ~14g
- Fiber: 0g

Cooking Time: 15-20 minutes

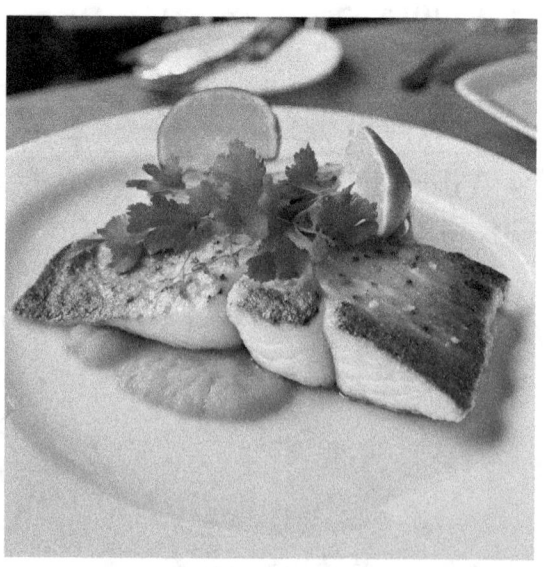

9. Catfish Creole

Ingredients:
- 4 catfish fillets (about 6 oz each)
- 2 tablespoons olive oil
- 1 onion, chopped
- 1 bell pepper, chopped
- 2 cloves garlic, minced
- 1 can (14 oz) diced tomatoes, undrained
- 1 teaspoon Creole seasoning
- Salt and pepper to taste
- Fresh parsley, chopped for garnish

Instructions:
1. Heat olive oil in a large skillet over medium heat. Add onion, bell pepper, and garlic; sauté until softened.
2. Stir in diced tomatoes and Creole seasoning. Bring to a simmer.
3. Season catfish fillets with salt and pepper, then nestle them into the skillet, spooning some sauce over the top.
4. Cover and simmer for 10-15 minutes or until the fish flakes easily with a fork.
5. Garnish with fresh parsley before serving.

Servings: 4

Nutritional Information (per serving):
- Calories: ~250
- Protein: ~35g
- Carbohydrates: ~8g
- Fat: ~10g
- Fiber: ~2g

Cooking Time: 25-30 minutes

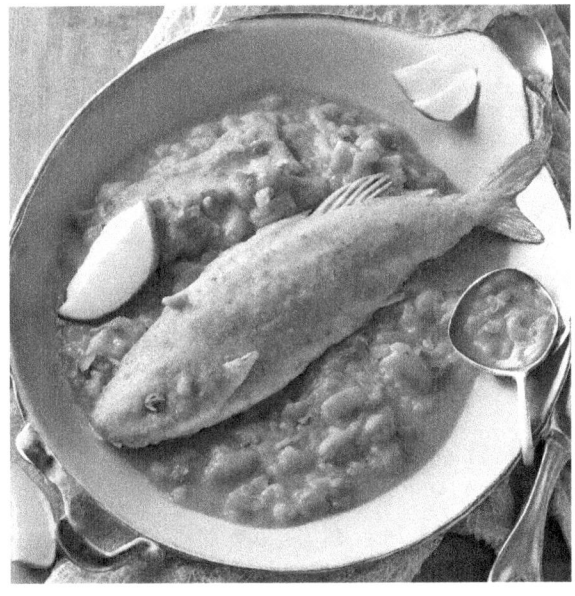

10. Oyster Stew

Ingredients:
- 12 oz fresh oysters, with their liquor
- 2 cups milk
- 1 cup heavy cream
- 4 tablespoons unsalted butter
- Salt and white pepper to taste
- Paprika for garnish
- Fresh chives, chopped for garnish

Instructions:
1. Melt butter in a saucepan over medium heat.
2. Add the oysters along with their liquor. Cook gently until the edges of the oysters curl.
3. Stir in milk and heavy cream, heating gently but do not boil.
4. Season with salt and white pepper.
5. Serve hot, garnished with paprika and chives.

Servings: 4

Nutritional Information (per serving):
- Calories: ~400
- Protein: ~10g
- Carbohydrates: ~8g
- Fat: ~35g
- Fiber: 0g

Cooking Time: 15-20 minutes

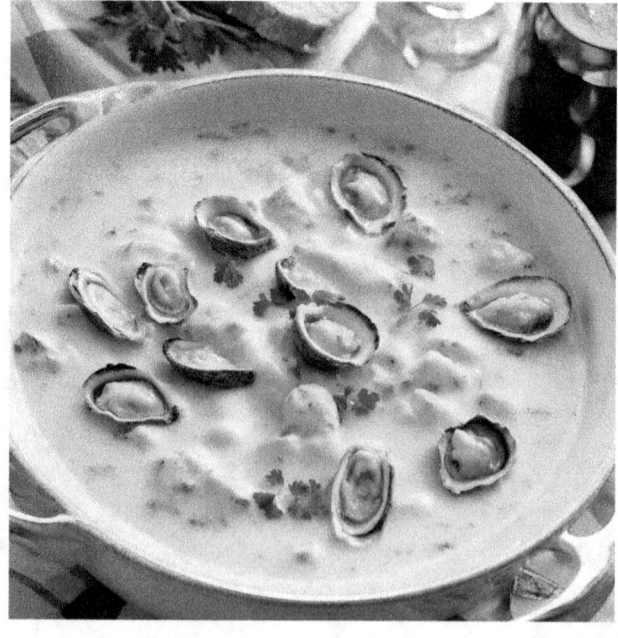

11. Salmon Mousse

Ingredients:
- 1 lb cooked salmon, flaked
- 1 envelope unflavored gelatin
- 1/4 cup cold water
- 1 cup mayonnaise
- 1 tablespoon lemon juice
- 2 tablespoons fresh dill, chopped
- Salt and white pepper to taste

Instructions:
1. Sprinkle gelatin over cold water in a small bowl; let stand for 5 minutes to soften.
2. Blend the cooked salmon, mayonnaise, lemon juice, dill, salt, and white pepper in a food processor until smooth.
3. Gently warm the gelatin mixture just until dissolved, then fold into the salmon mixture.
4. Pour into a mold or dish and refrigerate until set, at least 4 hours.
5. Unmold before serving, garnished with additional dill or lemon slices.

Servings: 6

Nutritional Information (per serving):
- Calories: ~350
- Protein: ~23g
- Carbohydrates: ~1g
- Fat: ~28g
- Fiber: 0g

Cooking Time: 4 hours 20 minutes (including setting time)

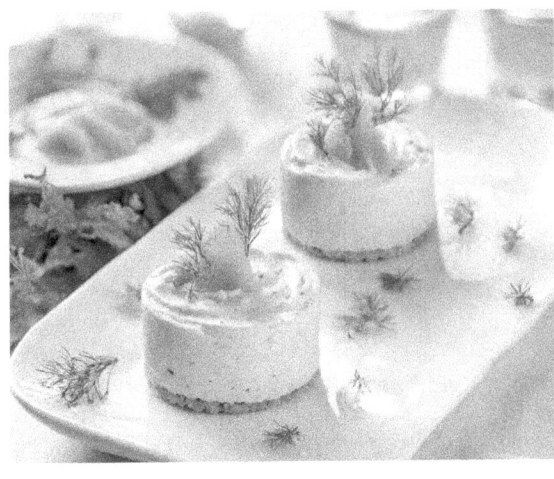

12. Trout Almondine

Ingredients:
- 4 trout fillets (about 6 oz each)
- 1/2 cup sliced almonds
- 4 tablespoons unsalted butter
- Juice of 1 lemon
- Salt and pepper to taste
- Fresh parsley, chopped for garnish

Instructions:
1. Season the trout fillets with salt and pepper.
2. Melt butter in a large skillet over medium heat. Add the trout, skin-side down, and cook until golden brown, about 3-4 minutes per side.
3. Remove the trout and keep warm. In the same skillet, add almonds and cook until golden.
4. Stir in lemon juice and pour the sauce over the trout.
5. Garnish with parsley and serve immediately.

Servings: 4

Nutritional Information (per serving):
- Calories: ~400
- Protein: ~35g
- Carbohydrates: ~3g
- Fat: ~28g
- Fiber: ~2g

Cooking Time: 15 minutes

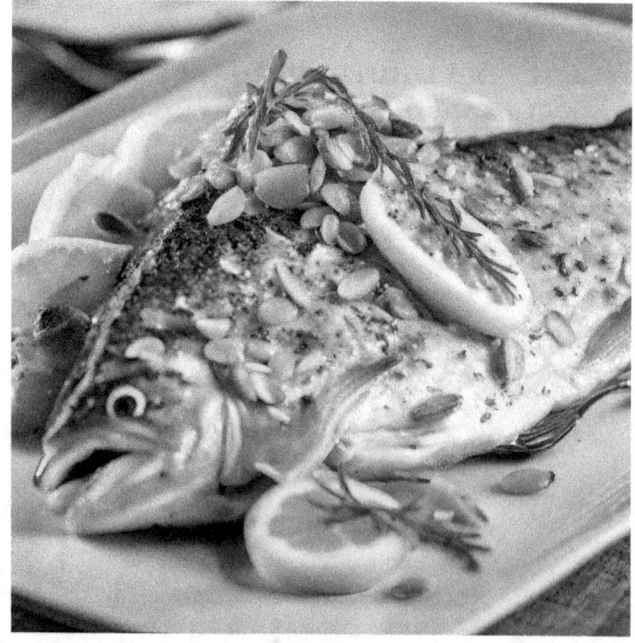

13. Grouper Piccata

Ingredients:
- 4 grouper fillets (about 6 oz each)
- 1/4 cup all-purpose flour
- 4 tablespoons unsalted butter
- 2 tablespoons olive oil
- Juice of 1 lemon
- 1/4 cup capers, rinsed
- 1/2 cup white wine
- Salt and pepper to taste
- Fresh parsley, chopped for garnish

Instructions:
1. Season the grouper fillets with salt and pepper, then dredge them lightly in flour, shaking off any excess.
2. In a large skillet, heat 2 tablespoons of butter and olive oil over medium-high heat. Add the fillets and cook until golden brown on each side and cooked through, about 3-4 minutes per side.
3. Remove the fillets from the skillet and keep warm. To the same skillet, add the white wine and lemon juice, scraping up any browned bits.
4. Reduce the sauce slightly, then stir in the capers and remaining butter until melted and the sauce has thickened.
5. Return the grouper to the skillet just to reheat, then transfer to serving plates.
6. Spoon the sauce over the fillets, garnish with fresh parsley, and serve immediately.

Servings: 4

Nutritional Information (per serving):
- Calories: ~350
- Protein: ~40g
- Carbohydrates: ~5g
- Fat: ~18g
- Fiber: ~0.5g

Cooking Time: 20 minutes

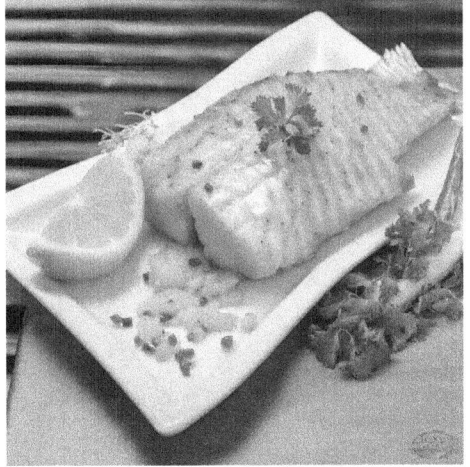

14. Sea Bass with Dill

Ingredients:
- 4 sea bass fillets (about 6 oz each)
- 2 tablespoons olive oil
- Salt and pepper to taste
- 1 lemon, sliced
- 2 tablespoons fresh dill, chopped
- 1/4 cup white wine or vegetable broth

Instructions:
1. Preheat the oven to 375°F (190°C).
2. Season the sea bass fillets with salt and pepper. Place them in a baking dish and drizzle with olive oil.
3. Arrange lemon slices over the fillets and sprinkle with dill.
4. Pour white wine or vegetable broth around the fillets in the dish.
5. Bake in the preheated oven until the fish flakes easily with a fork, about 15-20 minutes.
6. Serve hot, garnished with additional fresh dill if desired.

Servings: 4

Nutritional Information (per serving):
- Calories: ~280
- Protein: ~35g
- Carbohydrates: ~2g
- Fat: ~14g
- Fiber: ~0.5g

Cooking Time: 25 minutes

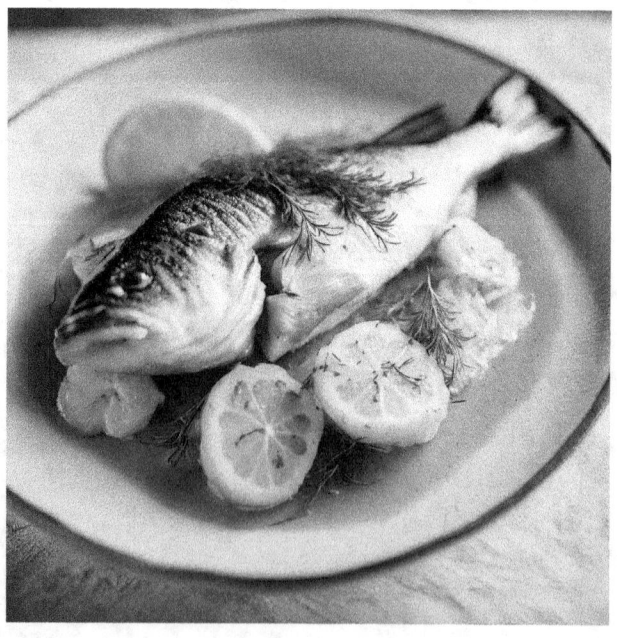

15. Prawn Stir-Fry

Ingredients:
- 1 lb prawns, peeled and deveined
- 2 tablespoons vegetable oil
- 1 bell pepper, sliced
- 1 onion, sliced
- 2 cloves garlic, minced
- 2 tablespoons soy sauce
- 1 tablespoon oyster sauce
- 1 teaspoon sesame oil
- Salt and pepper to taste
- Green onions, sliced for garnish

Instructions:
1. Heat the vegetable oil in a large skillet or wok over high heat.
2. Add the bell pepper, onion, and garlic, and stir-fry for 2-3 minutes until slightly softened.
3. Add the prawns and cook, stirring frequently, until they turn pink and are cooked through, about 3-5 minutes.
4. Stir in the soy sauce, oyster sauce, and sesame oil. Season with salt and pepper to taste.
5. Cook for another minute, ensuring everything is well coated and heated through.
6. Serve hot, garnished with sliced green onions.

Servings: 4

Nutritional Information (per serving):
- Calories: ~250
- Protein: ~25g
- Carbohydrates: ~6g
- Fat: ~14g
- Fiber: ~1g

Cooking Time: 15 minutes

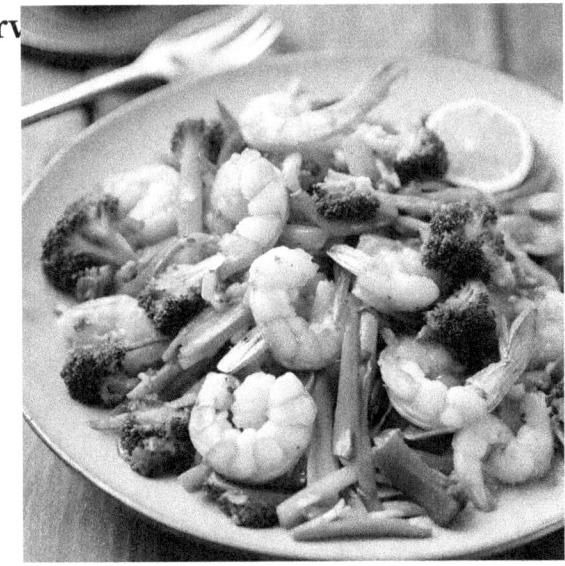

16. Sautéed Calamari

Ingredients:
- 4 grouper fillets (about 6 oz each)
- 1/4 cup all-purpose flour (for dusting)
- 4 tablespoons unsalted butter
- 2 tablespoons olive oil
- Juice of 1 lemon
- 1/4 cup capers, rinsed
- 1/2 cup chicken broth
- Salt and pepper to taste
- Fresh parsley, chopped for garnish

Instructions:
1. Season the grouper fillets with salt and pepper and lightly dust with flour.
2. Heat olive oil and 2 tablespoons of butter in a large skillet over medium-high heat. Add the fillets and cook until golden brown on both sides and cooked through, about 3-4 minutes per side. Remove the fish and set aside.
3. In the same skillet, add the lemon juice, capers, and chicken broth. Bring to a simmer, scraping up any browned bits from the bottom of the pan.
4. Reduce the sauce slightly, then whisk in the remaining butter until melted and the sauce has thickened.
5. Return the fish to the pan and coat with the sauce. Heat through gently.
6. Serve the fillets with the sauce poured over the top, garnished with fresh parsley.

Servings: 4

Nutritional Information (per serving):
- Calories: ~180
- Protein: ~18g
- Carbohydrates: ~3g
- Fat: ~10g
- Fiber: 0g

Cooking Time: 5-10 minutes

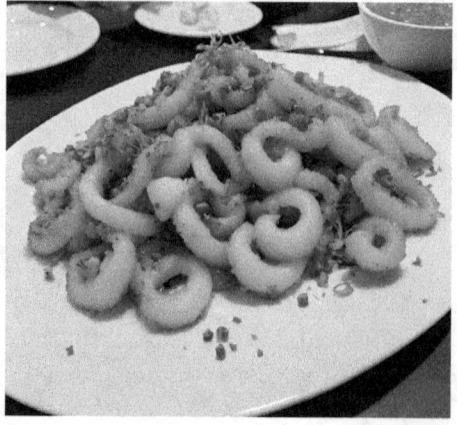

17. Grilled Mahi-Mahi

Ingredients:
- 4 mahi-mahi fillets (about 6 oz each)
- 2 tablespoons olive oil
- Juice of 1 lemon
- Salt and pepper to taste
- Lemon slices and fresh parsley for garnish

Instructions:
1. Preheat the grill to medium-high heat.
2. Brush both sides of the mahi-mahi fillets with olive oil and squeeze lemon juice over them. Season with salt and pepper.
3. Grill the fillets for about 4-5 minutes on each side, or until the fish flakes easily with a fork.
4. Serve hot, garnished with lemon slices and fresh parsley.

Servings: 4

Nutritional Information (per serving):
- Calories: ~200
- Protein: ~32g
- Carbohydrates: ~0g
- Fat: ~8g
- Fiber: 0g

Cooking Time: 10-15 minutes

18. Mussels Marinière

Ingredients:
- 2 lbs fresh mussels, cleaned and debearded
- 1 tablespoon butter
- 2 shallots, finely chopped
- 3 cloves garlic, minced
- 1 cup white wine
- Fresh parsley, chopped
- Salt and pepper to taste

Instructions:
1. In a large pot, melt the butter over medium heat. Add shallots and garlic, and sauté until soft.
2. Pour in the white wine, bring to a simmer.
3. Add the mussels, cover the pot, and let them steam for about 5-7 minutes until all the mussels have opened.
4. Discard any mussels that have not opened. Season with salt, pepper, and sprinkle with fresh parsley.
5. Serve hot with the broth.

Servings: 4

Nutritional Information (per serving):
- Calories: ~300
- Protein: ~24g
- Carbohydrates: ~10g
- Fat: ~10g
- Fiber: 0g

Cooking Time: 15-20 minutes

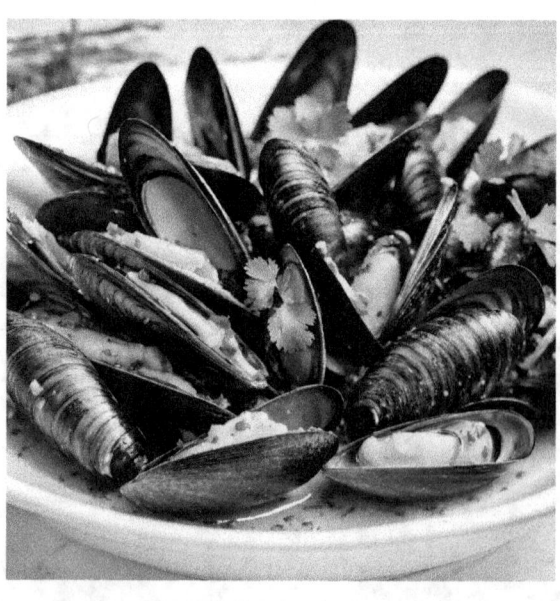

19. Lobster Bisque

Ingredients:
- 2 cooked lobsters, meat removed and shells reserved
- 2 tablespoons olive oil
- 1 onion, chopped
- 1 carrot, chopped
- 1 stalk celery, chopped
- 3 cloves garlic, minced
- 1/4 cup brandy (optional)
- 4 cups seafood or fish stock
- 1 cup heavy cream
- 2 tablespoons tomato paste
- Salt and cayenne pepper to taste
- Fresh parsley for garnish

Instructions:
1. In a large pot, heat olive oil over medium heat. Add lobster shells, onion, carrot, celery, and garlic. Sauté until vegetables are soft.
2. Deglaze with brandy if using, then add seafood stock and bring to a simmer.
3. Add tomato paste, simmer for 30 minutes.
4. Strain the soup, return the liquid to the pot. Add lobster meat and heavy cream, heat through.
5. Season with salt and cayenne pepper. Serve hot, garnished with fresh parsley.

Servings: 4

Nutritional Information (per serving):
- Calories: ~400
- Protein: ~20g
- Carbohydrates: ~10g
- Fat: ~30g
- Fiber: ~1g

Cooking Time: 50-60 minutes

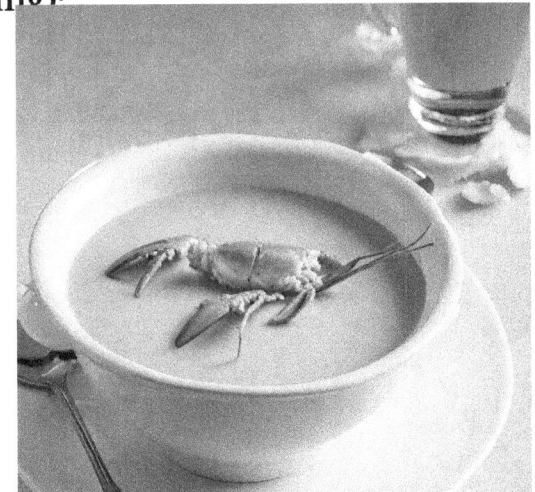

20. Haddock Chowder

Ingredients:
- 1 lb haddock fillets, cut into chunks
- 3 cups potatoes, diced
- 1 onion, chopped
- 2 cups milk
- 1 cup heavy cream
- 2 tablespoons butter
- Salt and pepper to taste
- Fresh parsley, chopped for garnish

Instructions:
1. In a large pot, melt butter over medium heat. Add onions and sauté until translucent.
2. Add potatoes and just enough water to cover them. Bring to a boil, then reduce heat and simmer until potatoes are tender.
3. Add haddock chunks, cook until the fish is opaque and flakes easily.
4. Stir in milk and heavy cream, heat through without boiling.
5. Season with salt and pepper. Serve hot, garnished with fresh parsley.

Servings: 4

Nutritional Information (per serving):
- Calories: ~450
- Protein: ~27g
- Carbohydrates: ~35g
- Fat: ~22g
- Fiber: ~3g

Cooking Time: 30-40 minutes

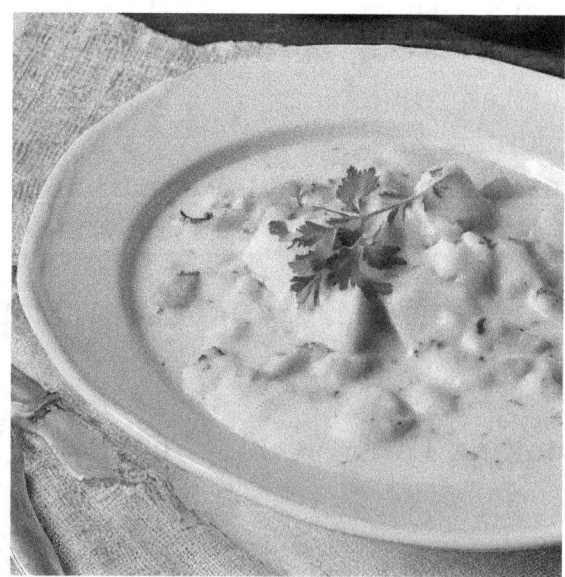

21. Tilapia in Parchment

Ingredients:
- 4 tilapia fillets
- Salt and pepper to taste
- 1 lemon, thinly sliced
- 4 sprigs of fresh thyme
- 4 tablespoons of olive oil
- 4 cloves of garlic, minced
- 4 tablespoons of dry white wine or chicken broth
- 4 sheets of parchment paper

Instructions:
1. Preheat your oven to 375°F (190°C).
2. Season each tilapia fillet with salt and pepper on both sides.
3. Place a tilapia fillet on each parchment paper sheet.
4. Top each fillet with lemon slices, thyme sprigs, minced garlic, and a tablespoon of olive oil.
5. Drizzle a tablespoon of white wine or chicken broth over each fillet.
6. Fold the parchment paper over the fish and crimp the edges tightly to create a sealed packet.
7. Place the packets on a baking sheet and bake in the preheated oven for 15-20 minutes, or until the fish is cooked through and flakes easily with a fork.
8. Carefully open the parchment packets and serve the tilapia hot.

Number of Serves: 4

Nutritional Information (per serving):
- Calories: 250
- Protein: 30g
- Carbohydrates: 3g
- Fat: 13g
- Fiber: 1g

Cooking Time: 15-20 minutes

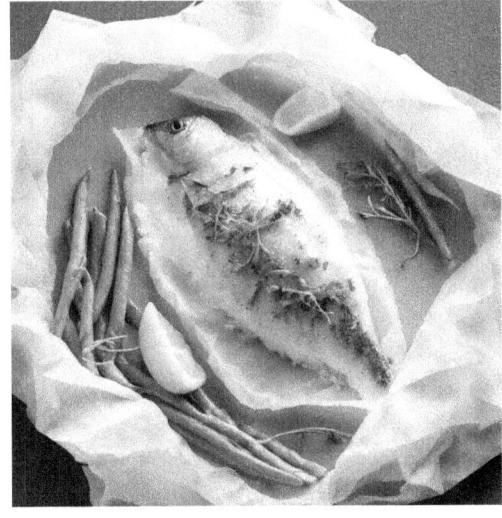

22. Broiled Scallops

Ingredients:
- 1 pound of scallops, rinsed and patted dry
- Salt and pepper to taste
- 2 tablespoons of olive oil
- 2 cloves of garlic, minced
- 2 tablespoons of chopped fresh parsley
- 1 lemon, juiced

Instructions:
1. Preheat the broiler on your oven.
2. Season the scallops with salt and pepper on both sides.
3. Arrange the scallops in a single layer on a broiler pan.
4. In a small bowl, mix together the olive oil, minced garlic, chopped parsley, and lemon juice.
5. Drizzle the olive oil mixture over the scallops.
6. Place the scallops under the preheated broiler and cook for 5-7 minutes, or until they are opaque and lightly browned on top.
7. Remove the scallops from the oven and serve immediately.

Number of Serves: 4

Nutritional Information (per serving):
- Calories: 150
- Protein: 20g
- Carbohydrates: 3g
- Fat: 7g
- Fiber: 0g

Cooking Time: 5-7 minutes

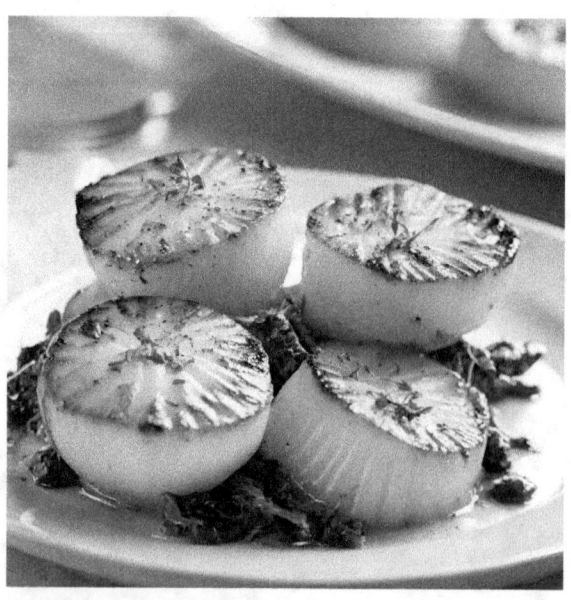

23. Flounder Meunière

Ingredients:
- 4 flounder fillets
- Salt and pepper to taste
- ½ cup of all-purpose flour
- 4 tablespoons of unsalted butter
- 2 tablespoons of olive oil
- 2 tablespoons of freshly squeezed lemon juice
- 2 tablespoons of chopped fresh parsley
- Lemon wedges for serving

Instructions:
1. Season the flounder fillets with salt and pepper on both sides.
2. Dredge the fillets in flour, shaking off any excess.
3. In a large skillet, heat the butter and olive oil over medium-high heat until the butter begins to foam.
4. Carefully add the flounder fillets to the skillet and cook for 2-3 minutes per side, or until they are golden brown and cooked through.
5. Transfer the cooked fillets to a serving platter.
6. Add the lemon juice and chopped parsley to the skillet, swirling to combine.
7. Pour the sauce over the flounder fillets.
8. Serve the flounder meunière hot with lemon wedges on the side.

Number of Serves: 4

Nutritional Information (per serving):
- Calories: 300
- Protein: 25g
- Carbohydrates: 10g
- Fat: 17g
- Fiber: 1g

Cooking Time: 6-8 minutes

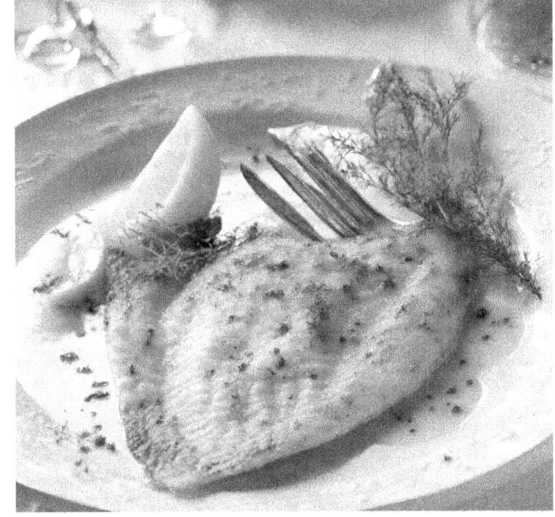

DESSERTS

1. Zabaglione

Ingredients:
- 4 large egg yolks
- ¼ cup sugar
- ½ cup Marsala wine (or any sweet wine)
- Fresh berries for serving (optional)

Instructions:
1. In a heatproof bowl, whisk together the egg yolks and sugar until pale and creamy.
2. Place the bowl over a pot of simmering water, making sure the bottom of the bowl doesn't touch the water.
3. Slowly whisk in the Marsala wine and continue whisking constantly until the mixture thickens and triples in volume, about 5-7 minutes.
4. Remove from heat and serve immediately, either on its own or over fresh berries.

Number of Serves: 4

Nutritional Information (per serving):
- Calories: 190
- Protein: 4g
- Carbohydrates: 19g
- Fat: 9g
- Fiber: 0g

Cooking Time: 5-7 minutes

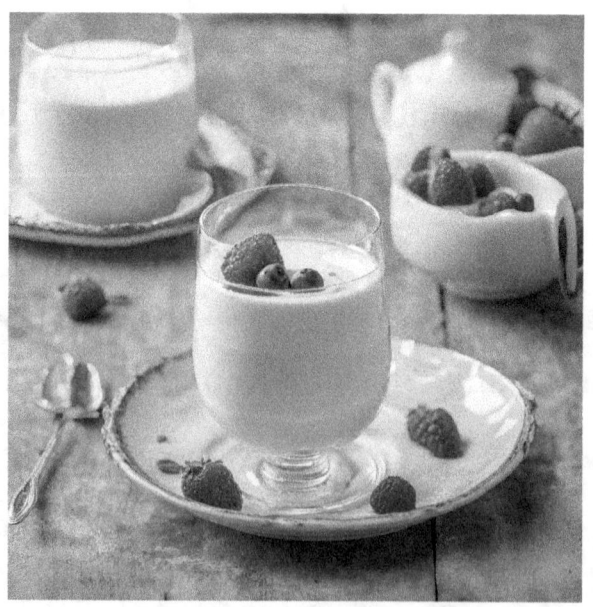

2. Apple Crisp

Ingredients:
- 4 cups sliced apples
- 2 tablespoons lemon juice
- ½ cup rolled oats
- ¼ cup all-purpose flour
- ¼ cup brown sugar
- ¼ teaspoon ground cinnamon
- 3 tablespoons unsalted butter, melted

Instructions:
1. Preheat your oven to 350°F (175°C).
2. In a bowl, toss the sliced apples with lemon juice and place them in a baking dish.
3. In another bowl, mix together the rolled oats, flour, brown sugar, cinnamon, and melted butter until crumbly.
4. Sprinkle the oat mixture evenly over the apples.
5. Bake in the preheated oven for 30-35 minutes, or until the topping is golden brown and the apples are tender.
6. Serve warm.

Number of Serves: 4

Nutritional Information (per serving):
- Calories: 220
- Protein: 2g
- Carbohydrates: 38g
- Fat: 8g
- Fiber: 4g

Cooking Time: 30-35 minutes

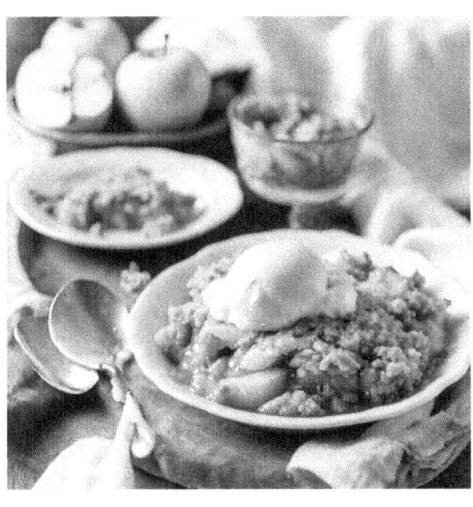

3. Milky Semolina Pudding

Ingredients:
- 4 cups milk
- ½ cup semolina
- ¼ cup sugar (adjust to taste)
- 1 teaspoon vanilla extract
- Pinch of salt
- Ground cinnamon or nutmeg for garnish (optional)

Instructions:
1. In a saucepan, bring the milk to a gentle simmer over medium heat.
2. Gradually whisk in the semolina, sugar, vanilla extract, and salt.
3. Cook, stirring constantly, for about 5-7 minutes, or until the mixture thickens to a pudding-like consistency.
4. Remove from heat and let it cool slightly.
5. Serve warm or chilled, garnished with ground cinnamon or nutmeg if desired.

Number of Serves: 4

Nutritional Information (per serving):
- Calories: 240
- Protein: 9g
- Carbohydrates: 35g
- Fat: 6g
- Fiber: 1g

Cooking Time: 5-7 minutes

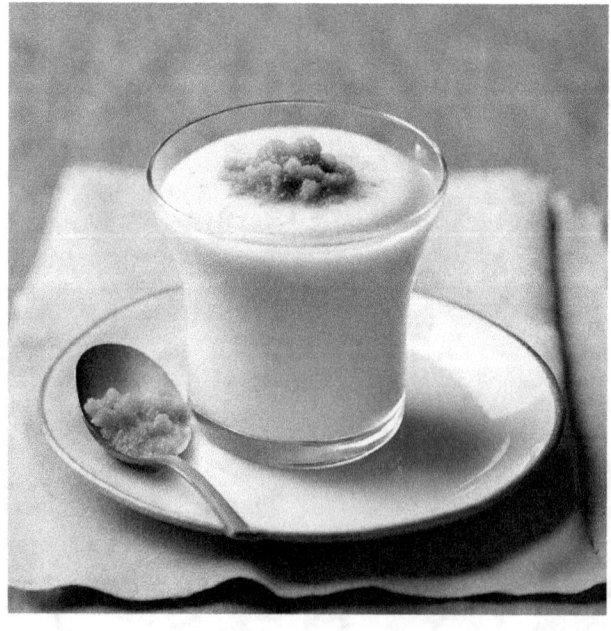

4. Simple Poached Quince

Ingredients:
- 4 quinces, peeled, cored, and quartered
- 4 cups water
- 1 cup sugar
- 1 cinnamon stick
- 2 cloves
- Zest of 1 lemon

Instructions:
1. In a large saucepan, combine water, sugar, cinnamon stick, cloves, and lemon zest. Bring to a boil.
2. Add the quince quarters to the boiling syrup.
3. Reduce heat to low, cover, and simmer for about 1-1.5 hours, or until the quinces are tender.
4. Remove the quince quarters from the syrup and serve warm or chilled.
5. Optionally, you can reduce the syrup further by boiling until thickened and serve it alongside the poached quinces.

Number of Serves: 4

Nutritional Information (per serving):
- Calories: 210
- Protein: 1g
- Carbohydrates: 55g
- Fat: 0g
- Fiber: 5g

Cooking Time: 1-1.5 hours

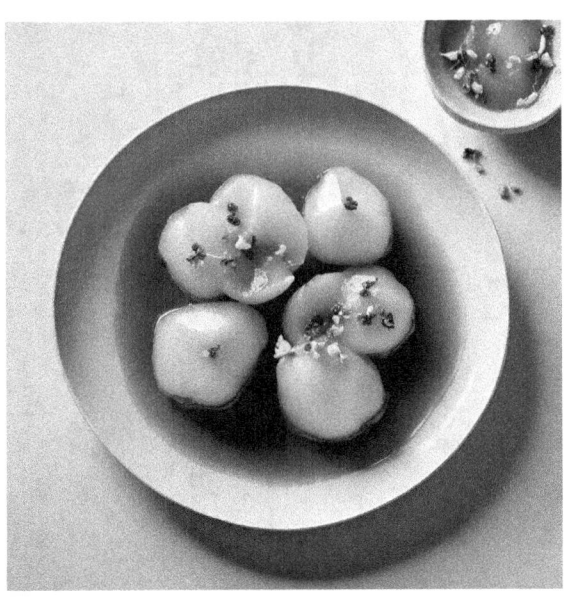

5. Yogurt Parfait

Ingredients:
- 2 cups plain yogurt
- 1 cup granola
- 1 cup mixed fresh berries (such as strawberries, blueberries, raspberries)
- 2 tablespoons honey or maple syrup (optional)

Instructions:
1. In serving glasses or bowls, layer the yogurt, granola, and mixed berries.
2. Repeat the layers until all ingredients are used, finishing with a layer of berries on top.
3. Drizzle honey or maple syrup over the top if desired.
4. Serve immediately or refrigerate until ready to serve.

Number of Serves: 2

Nutritional Information (per serving):
- Calories: 300
- Protein: 10g
- Carbohydrates: 50g
- Fat: 7g
- Fiber: 6g

No Cooking Required

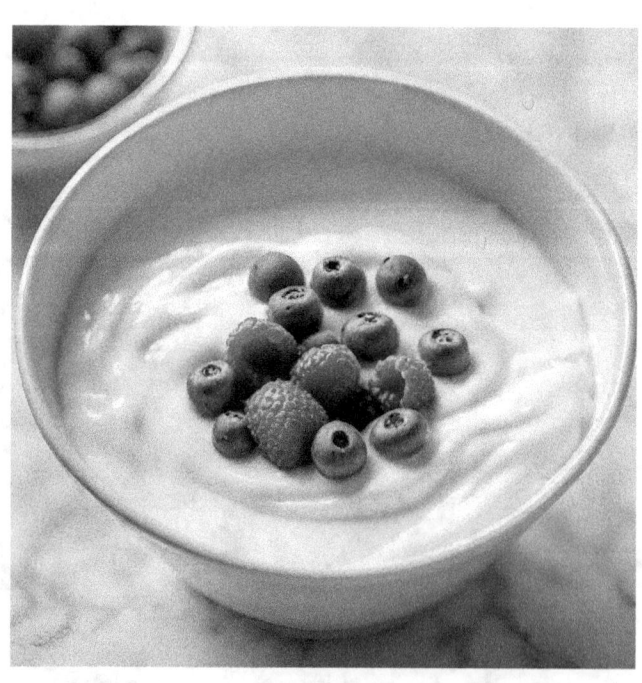

6. Lemon Sponge Cake

Ingredients:
- 1 cup all-purpose flour
- 1 teaspoon baking powder
- ½ teaspoon salt
- ½ cup unsalted butter, softened
- 1 cup granulated sugar
- 2 large eggs
- ½ cup milk
- Zest of 1 lemon
- Juice of 1 lemon
- Powdered sugar for dusting (optional)

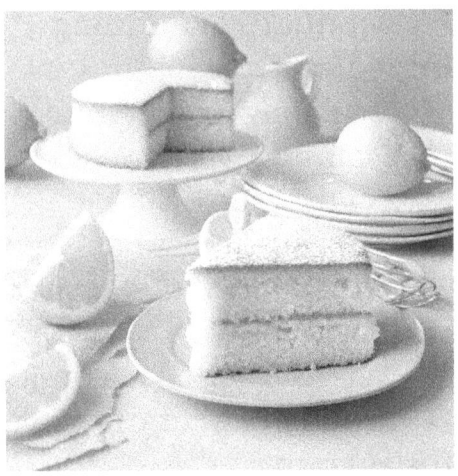

Instructions:
1. Preheat your oven to 350°F (175°C). Grease and flour a 9-inch round cake pan.
2. In a medium bowl, sift together the flour, baking powder, and salt.
3. In a separate bowl, cream together the butter and sugar until light and fluffy.
4. Beat in the eggs, one at a time, then stir in the lemon zest and lemon juice.
5. Gradually mix in the dry ingredients alternately with the milk until just combined.
6. Pour the batter into the prepared cake pan and smooth the top.
7. Bake in the preheated oven for 25-30 minutes, or until a toothpick inserted into the center comes out clean.
8. Allow the cake to cool in the pan for 10 minutes before transferring to a wire rack to cool completely.
9. Dust with powdered sugar before serving if desired.

Number of Serves: 8

Nutritional Information (per serving):
- Calories: 250
- Protein: 4g
- Carbohydrates: 35g
- Fat: 11g
- Fiber: 1g

Cooking Time: 25-30 minutes

7. Coconut Rice Pudding

Ingredients:
- 1 cup long-grain white rice
- 2 cups coconut milk
- 2 cups water
- ⅓ cup sugar
- ½ teaspoon vanilla extract
- Pinch of salt
- ¼ cup shredded coconut (optional, for garnish)
- Ground cinnamon for garnish (optional)

Instructions:
1. In a saucepan, combine the rice, coconut milk, water, sugar, vanilla extract, and salt.
2. Bring the mixture to a boil over medium heat, then reduce the heat to low.
3. Simmer, uncovered, stirring occasionally, for about 20-25 minutes, or until the rice is tender and the mixture has thickened.
4. Remove from heat and let it cool slightly.
5. Serve warm or chilled, garnished with shredded coconut and ground cinnamon if desired.

Number of Serves: 4

Nutritional Information (per serving):
- Calories: 300
- Protein: 3g
- Carbohydrates: 45g
- Fat: 12g
- Fiber: 2g

Cooking Time: 20-25 minutes

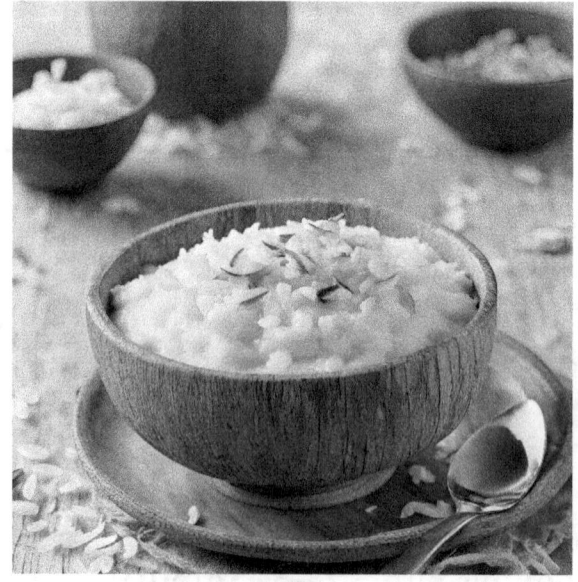

8. Bread Pudding

Ingredients:
- 4 cups cubed stale bread (such as French bread or brioche)
- 2 cups milk
- 2 large eggs
- ½ cup sugar
- 1 teaspoon vanilla extract
- ½ teaspoon ground cinnamon
- ¼ teaspoon ground nutmeg
- ¼ cup raisins (optional)
- Whipped cream or vanilla ice cream for serving (optional)

Instructions:
1. Preheat your oven to 350°F (175°C). Grease a baking dish.
2. In a large bowl, whisk together the milk, eggs, sugar, vanilla extract, cinnamon, and nutmeg until well combined.
3. Add the cubed bread and raisins (if using) to the bowl, stirring until the bread is evenly coated.
4. Let the mixture sit for about 15-20 minutes, allowing the bread to absorb the liquid.
5. Pour the bread mixture into the prepared baking dish.
6. Bake in the preheated oven for 40-45 minutes, or until the pudding is set and the top is golden brown.
7. Serve warm with whipped cream or vanilla ice cream if desired.

Number of Serves: 6

Nutritional Information (per serving):
- Calories: 300
- Protein: 8g
- Carbohydrates: 45g
- Fat: 10g
- Fiber: 2g

Cooking Time: 40-45 minutes

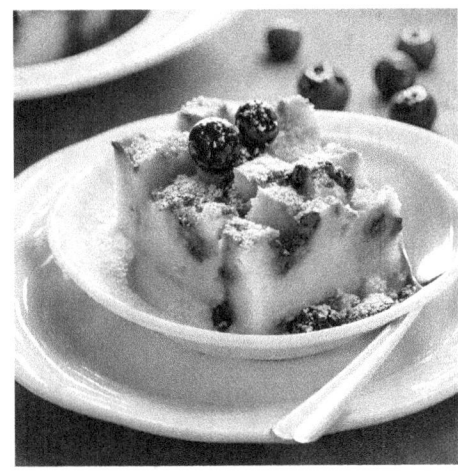

9. Vanilla Panna Cotta

Ingredients:
- 2 cups heavy cream
- ½ cup milk
- ¼ cup sugar
- 1 teaspoon vanilla extract
- 2 teaspoons unflavored gelatin
- 2 tablespoons cold water
- Fresh berries or fruit compote for serving (optional)

Instructions:
1. In a saucepan, combine the heavy cream, milk, sugar, and vanilla extract. Heat over medium heat until the mixture just begins to simmer, stirring occasionally.
2. While the cream mixture is heating, sprinkle the gelatin over the cold water in a small bowl. Let it sit for about 5 minutes to soften.
3. Remove the cream mixture from heat and stir in the softened gelatin until completely dissolved.
4. Pour the mixture into serving glasses or molds.
5. Refrigerate for at least 4 hours, or until set.
6. Serve chilled, topped with fresh berries or fruit compote if desired.

Number of Serves: 4

Nutritional Information (per serving):
- Calories: 350
- Protein: 4g
- Carbohydrates: 15g
- Fat: 30g
- Fiber: 0g

Cooking Time: 10 minutes (plus chilling time)

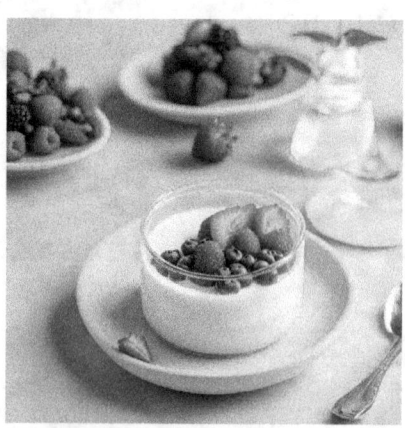

8-WEEK MEAL PLAN

Week 1

Day 1:
- **Breakfast:** Scrambled eggs with white toast and margarine.
- **Lunch:** Chicken rice soup with saltine crackers.
- **Dinner:** Baked salmon, mashed potatoes (no skins), and steamed carrots.
- **Snacks:** Applesauce, low-fat yogurt.

Day 2:
- **Breakfast:** Oatmeal (well-cooked) with banana slices.
- **Lunch:** Turkey sandwich on white bread with a side of boiled green beans.
- **Dinner:** Grilled chicken breast, white rice, and stewed zucchini.
- **Snacks:** Gelatin, peach slices (canned in water).

Day 3:
- **Breakfast:** Pancakes with maple syrup, a side of canned pears.
- **Lunch:** Cream of potato soup, white rolls with margarine.
- **Dinner:** Beef stew (lean cuts of beef, potatoes, carrots), white bread.
- **Snacks:** Vanilla pudding, crackers.

Day 4:
- **Breakfast:** French toast with a small amount of strawberry jam.
- **Lunch:** Baked cod, white pasta with olive oil, steamed spinach (small amount).
- **Dinner:** Roast turkey, squash puree, rice pilaf.
- **Snacks:** Apple sauce, graham crackers.

Day 5:
- **Breakfast:** Bagel (plain or egg) with cream cheese.
- **Lunch:** Chicken noodle soup, white bread with margarine.
- **Dinner:** Pork loin, sweet potatoes (mashed), boiled peas.
- **Snacks:** Cottage cheese (low-fat), canned mandarin oranges.

Day 6:
- **Breakfast:** Cream of wheat, slices of melon.
- **Lunch:** Egg salad sandwich on white bread, cucumber slices.
- **Dinner:** Baked chicken, couscous, steamed asparagus tips.
- **Snacks:** Yogurt, saltine crackers.

Day 7:
- **Breakfast:** Soft boiled eggs, white toast with butter, and honey.
- **Lunch:** Tuna salad (light on mayonnaise) on white bread, soft-cooked carrots.
- **Dinner:** Spaghetti with ground turkey sauce, steamed broccoli florets.
- **Snacks:** Rice cakes, banana.

Week 2

Day 1:
- **Breakfast:** Banana smoothie made with low-fat yogurt.
- **Lunch:** Grilled cheese sandwich on white bread, cream of asparagus soup.
- **Dinner:** Turkey meatloaf, mashed butternut squash, steamed green beans.
- **Snacks:** Rice pudding, pretzels.

Day 2:
- **Breakfast:** Soft-boiled egg, white toast with avocado spread.
- **Lunch:** Lentil soup (well-cooked lentils), white pita bread.
- **Dinner:** Baked tilapia, quinoa, roasted carrots.
- **Snacks:** Baked apple, digestive biscuits.

Day 3:
- **Breakfast:** Yogurt with honey and sliced peaches.
- **Lunch:** Chicken caesar salad (with well-cooked chicken and light dressing), white bread croutons.
- **Dinner:** Beef tenderloin, oven-roasted potatoes, pureed peas.
- **Snacks:** Gelatin with whipped topping, low-fiber cereal bars.

Day 4:
- **Breakfast:** Porridge with maple syrup and blueberries.
- **Lunch:** Baked sweet potato with cottage cheese topping, boiled spinach.
- **Dinner:** Roasted chicken with gravy, couscous, steamed mixed vegetables (carrots, zucchini).
- **Snacks:** Custard, saltines with cheese spread.

Day 5:
- **Breakfast:** Pancakes with honey and a side of canned fruit cocktail.
- **Lunch:** Tuna melt sandwich on white bread, vegetable soup (strained).
- **Dinner:** Spaghetti with meatballs, tomato sauce (smooth), steamed broccoli.
- **Snacks:** Apple sauce, vanilla yogurt.

Day 6:
- **Breakfast:** Scrambled eggs with cheese, white toast with jam.
- **Lunch:** Roast beef sandwich on white roll, lettuce and tomato, mashed avocado.
- **Dinner:** Grilled shrimp, white rice, pureed butternut squash.
- **Snacks:** Pears (canned in juice), crackers with peanut butter.

Day 7:
- **Breakfast:** Bagel with light cream cheese and jelly.
- **Lunch:** Quiche Lorraine (no crust), steamed carrots.
- **Dinner:** Lemon-baked cod, polenta, steamed asparagus (tips only).
- **Snacks:** Greek yogurt, rice cakes.

Week 3

For Week 3, introduce slightly more fiber while still focusing on well-tolerated foods, aiming for nutritional balance and variety.

Day 1:
- **Breakfast:** Muesli (soaked overnight in milk), banana.
- **Lunch:** BLT sandwich on white bread (lightly toasted), cucumber salad.
- **Dinner:** Chicken stir-fry (with bell peppers, snap peas, and a mild sauce), jasmine rice.
- **Snacks:** Peach slices, oatmeal cookies.

Day 2:
- **Breakfast:** French toast with apple compote.
- **Lunch:** Salmon salad (with light mayo) on white bread, beetroot salad (small portion).
- **Dinner:** Roast pork with applesauce, mashed sweet potatoes, green peas.
- **Snacks:** Fruit yogurt, ginger snaps.

Day 3:
- **Breakfast:** Omelet with cheese and ham, white toast.
- **Lunch:** Vegetable lasagna (with spinach and ricotta), caesar salad (no croutons).
- **Dinner:** Baked haddock with lemon butter, barley, steamed kale.
- **Snacks:** Cottage cheese with canned pineapple, plain crackers.

Day 4:
- **Breakfast:** Smoothie with papaya, mango, and low-fat milk.
- **Lunch:** Chicken and avocado wrap (in a soft tortilla), tomato soup.
- **Dinner:** Beef bourguignon (with tender vegetables), mashed potatoes.
- **Snacks:** Melon slices, cheese sticks.

Day 5:
- **Breakfast:** Porridge with sliced strawberries and almond slices.
- **Lunch:** Shrimp pasta salad (with olive oil and lemon dressing), arugula salad.
- **Dinner:** Turkey chili (mild, with well-cooked beans), cornbread.
- **Snacks:** Applesauce, pretzel sticks.

Day 6:
- **Breakfast:** Yogurt with granola and raspberries.
- **Lunch:** Egg salad on soft whole wheat bread, side of steamed mixed veggies.
- **Dinner:** Pan-seared duck breast, wild rice, sautéed spinach (very well cooked).
- **Snacks:** Baked pear, graham crackers with cream cheese.

Day 7:
- **Breakfast:** Smoothie bowl with blended banana, spinach (for color, not texture), and mango, topped with a few sliced almonds.
- **Lunch:** Quinoa salad with cucumber, tomatoes, feta cheese, and a light vinaigrette.
- **Dinner:** Lamb chops, roasted parsnips, and puréed carrots.
- **Snacks:** Canned peaches, vanilla pudding.

Week 4

In Week 4, continue to maintain a variety with a slight increase in fiber and texture, ensuring foods are still easily digestible and well-tolerated.

Day 1:
- **Breakfast:** Oat pancakes with maple syrup and a side of kiwi slices.
- **Lunch:** Chicken gyro in a soft pita, side of Greek yogurt with cucumber.
- **Dinner:** Grilled sea bass, orzo with light olive oil, roasted bell peppers (peeled).
- **Snacks:** Watermelon slices, low-fat cheese slices.

Day 2:
- **Breakfast:** Avocado toast on sourdough (ensure the bread is not too crusty), poached egg.
- **Lunch:** Beef stew with soft-cooked veggies and potatoes, side of white bread.
- **Dinner:** Pasta primavera with chicken (ensure vegetables are well-cooked and soft).
- **Snacks:** Cottage cheese with soft peach slices, rice crackers.

Day 3:
- **Breakfast:** Fruit salad (melon, banana, and berries), cottage cheese.
- **Lunch:** Tuna pasta salad with sweetcorn, cucumber, and a light mayo dressing.
- **Dinner:** Roasted chicken thighs, quinoa salad with roasted pumpkin (soft).
- **Snacks:** Apple sauce, oat biscuits.

Day 4:
- **Breakfast:** Scrambled tofu with turmeric, on a soft whole grain roll.
- **Lunch:** Chicken and sweet potato soup, soft dinner roll.
- **Dinner:** Grilled trout, creamy polenta, steamed green beans.
- **Snacks:** Mango slices, wheat crackers with hummus.

Day 5:
- **Breakfast:** Whole grain waffles with yogurt and honey.
- **Lunch:** Caprese salad (tomato, mozzarella, basil) with balsamic reduction, side of sourdough bread.
- **Dinner:** Pork tenderloin, roasted sweet potato wedges, asparagus tips.
- **Snacks:** Kiwi slices, popcorn (without hulls).

Day 6:
- **Breakfast:** Berry smoothie with protein powder, spinach, and oat milk.
- **Lunch:** Turkey and cranberry sauce sandwich on soft whole wheat bread, lettuce.
- **Dinner:** Sautéed shrimp, couscous with parsley, roasted zucchini (skin removed).
- **Snacks:** Pudding, saltine crackers with jelly.

Day 7:
- **Breakfast:** Baked oatmeal with apples and cinnamon.
- **Lunch:** Vegetable quiche (made with low-fiber vegetables like zucchini, tomato, and eggplant), green salad.
- **Dinner:** Stuffed bell peppers (with ground turkey and rice, ensure the pepper is cooked until very soft).
- **Snacks:** Banana, soft granola bars.

Week 5

Day 1:
- **Breakfast:** Scrambled eggs with soft-cooked spinach and white toast.
- **Lunch:** Turkey and cheese roll-up with soft tortilla, side of mashed carrots.
- **Dinner:** Grilled tilapia, jasmine rice, steamed broccoli florets.
- **Snacks:** Banana, low-fat yogurt.

Day 2:
- **Breakfast:** Oatmeal with sliced strawberries and almond milk.
- **Lunch:** Quinoa salad with avocado, cherry tomatoes, and diced chicken breast.
- **Dinner:** Baked chicken breast, sweet potato puree, green beans.
- **Snacks:** Applesauce, whole grain crackers.

Day 3:
- **Breakfast:** Smoothie with blueberries, spinach, banana, and oat milk.
- **Lunch:** Soft whole wheat pasta with olive oil and Parmesan, steamed zucchini.
- **Dinner:** Roast beef, quinoa, and steamed carrots.
- **Snacks:** Peach slices, cottage cheese.

Day 4:
- **Breakfast:** Pancakes with maple syrup and a side of canned peaches.
- **Lunch:** Chicken noodle soup with soft vegetables, white bread roll.
- **Dinner:** Baked cod with lemon, mashed potatoes, peas.
- **Snacks:** Rice pudding, graham crackers.

Day 5:
- **Breakfast:** French toast with a dab of butter and syrup, side of mandarin oranges.
- **Lunch:** BLT wrap with turkey bacon in a soft tortilla, side of butternut squash soup.
- **Dinner:** Pork tenderloin, couscous, steamed spinach.
- **Snacks:** Gelatin dessert, vanilla yogurt.

Day 6:
- **Breakfast:** Cream of wheat with honey and milk.
- **Lunch:** Tuna salad on soft whole grain bread, cucumber slices.
- **Dinner:** Turkey meatballs in marinara sauce, spaghetti, steamed broccoli.
- **Snacks:** Apple sauce, cheese slices.

Day 7:
- **Breakfast:** Bagel with light cream cheese and jelly.
- **Lunch:** Grilled cheese sandwich on sourdough, tomato soup.
- **Dinner:** Lemon-herb chicken, roasted butternut squash, green beans.
- **Snacks:** Pears (canned in juice), plain yogurt.

Week 6

Day 1:
- **Breakfast:** Mashed avocado on white toast, poached egg.
- **Lunch:** Lentil soup with soft carrots, side of white rice.
- **Dinner:** Grilled salmon, wild rice, steamed asparagus tips.
- **Snacks:** Baked apple, low-fat yogurt.

Day 2:
- **Breakfast:** Banana smoothie with peanut butter and almond milk.
- **Lunch:** Egg salad sandwich on soft whole wheat bread, boiled beets.
- **Dinner:** Chicken stir-fry with bell peppers and snap peas, jasmine rice.
- **Snacks:** Cottage cheese, canned pineapple.

Day 3:
- **Breakfast:** Oatmeal with maple syrup and sliced bananas.
- **Lunch:** Quiche with soft vegetables (zucchini, tomato), green salad.
- **Dinner:** Beef stew with potatoes and carrots, soft dinner roll.
- **Snacks:** Melon slices, graham crackers.

Day 4:
- **Breakfast:** Scrambled eggs with soft whole grain toast, side of honeydew melon.
- **Lunch:** Tuna wrap in a soft tortilla, side of mashed sweet potatoes.
- **Dinner:** Baked trout, polenta, steamed mixed vegetables.
- **Snacks:** Apple sauce, whole grain crackers.

Day 5:
- **Breakfast:** Greek yogurt with honey and soft granola.
- **Lunch:** Chicken Caesar salad with soft croutons, Caesar dressing.
- **Dinner:** Pork loin roast, mashed potatoes, peas.
- **Snacks:** Peach slices, rice cakes.

Day 6:
- **Breakfast:** Smoothie with mixed berries, spinach, and yogurt.
- **Lunch:** Soft whole wheat pasta with Alfredo sauce and steamed broccoli.
- **Dinner:** Grilled chicken breast, couscous, steamed carrots.
- **Snacks:** Gelatin dessert, vanilla pudding.

Day 7:
- **Breakfast:** French toast with banana slices and a small amount of syrup.
- **Lunch:** Baked sweet potato topped with black beans (ensure they are well-cooked) and cheese.
- **Dinner:** Shrimp risotto, roasted zucchini (make sure it's soft).
- **Snacks:** Canned peaches, low-fat cottage cheese.

Week 7

Day 1:
- **Breakfast:** Chia seed pudding with almond milk and kiwi slices.
- **Lunch:** Turkey and Swiss cheese sandwich on soft whole grain bread, side of carrot soup.
- **Dinner:** Baked haddock, barley, steamed snap peas.
- **Snacks:** Yogurt with mashed raspberries, saltine crackers.

Day 2:
- **Breakfast:** Smoothie with avocado, pear, and spinach.
- **Lunch:** Quinoa and black bean salad (ensure beans are soft), small side of guacamole.
- **Dinner:** Lemon garlic chicken, mashed cauliflower, steamed green beans.
- **Snacks:** Apple sauce, wheat thins.

Day 3:
- **Breakfast:** Pancakes with blueberries and whipped cream.
- **Lunch:** Lentil and vegetable stew, soft whole wheat roll.
- **Dinner:** Grilled pork chops, sweet potato fries, kale salad (ensure kale is tender).
- **Snacks:** Banana, low-fat cheese sticks.

Day 4:
- **Breakfast:** Oatmeal with diced apples and cinnamon.
- **Lunch:** Chicken gyro in a soft pita, side of cucumber salad.
- **Dinner:** Beef stir-fry with bell peppers and onions, served over soft-cooked noodles.
- **Snacks:** Mandarin oranges, vanilla yogurt.

Day 5:
- **Breakfast:** Scrambled tofu with turmeric, on soft whole grain toast.
- **Lunch:** Baked cod with a side of mashed peas and carrots.
- **Dinner:** Turkey meatloaf, quinoa, steamed broccoli.
- **Snacks:** Pears (canned in juice), rice crackers.

Day 6:
- **Breakfast:** Greek yogurt with sliced peaches and a drizzle of honey.
- **Lunch:** Avocado and shrimp salad with light dressing, soft dinner roll.
- **Dinner:** Chicken parmesan (with soft breading) over spaghetti, side of steamed spinach.
- **Snacks:** Cottage cheese, soft granola bars.

Day 7:
- **Breakfast:** Bagel with light cream cheese and smoked salmon.
- **Lunch:** Soft whole grain wrap with hummus, turkey breast, and roasted bell peppers.
- **Dinner:** Salmon fillet with a dill cream sauce, wild rice, roasted butternut squash (ensure softness).
- **Snacks:** Gelatin with fruit, saltines with cheese spread.

Week 8

Day 1:
- **Breakfast:** Soft-boiled eggs, avocado slices, white toast.
- **Lunch:** Chicken and rice soup, soft breadsticks.
- **Dinner:** Grilled tilapia, orzo pasta salad with olives and feta, steamed asparagus.
- **Snacks:** Apple slices, almond butter.

Day 2:
- **Breakfast:** Smoothie with mango, coconut milk, and protein powder.
- **Lunch:** Spinach and feta stuffed chicken breast, couscous, boiled carrots.
- **Dinner:** Spaghetti squash with marinara sauce and meatballs, steamed green beans.
- **Snacks:** Yogurt with granola, cucumber slices.

Day 3:
- **Breakfast:** Banana and peanut butter on soft whole grain bread.
- **Lunch:** Beef and barley soup, white dinner roll.
- **Dinner:** Baked lemon pepper chicken, mashed potatoes, peas.
- **Snacks:** Rice pudding, crackers with cheese.

Day 4:
- **Breakfast:** Toasted bagel with cream cheese and smoked salmon.
- **Lunch:** Tuna melt on sourdough, side of cucumber salad.
- **Dinner:** Pork stir-fry with bell peppers and onions, brown rice.
- **Snacks:** Apple sauce, graham crackers with peanut butter.

Day 5:
- **Breakfast:** Waffles with maple syrup and a side of canned peaches.
- **Lunch:** Spinach and ricotta stuffed pasta shells, marinara sauce, soft dinner roll.
- **Dinner:** Lemon herb roasted chicken, mashed potatoes, steamed peas.
- **Snacks:** Cottage cheese, fresh pineapple.

FOOD TRAKER JOURNAL

DATE:

MON	BREAKFAST	DINNER
	LUNCH	SNACK
TUE	BREAKFAST	DINNER
	LUNCH	SNACK
WED	BREAKFAST	DINNER
	LUNCH	SNACK
THUR	BREAKFAST	DINNER
	LUNCH	SNACK
FRI	BREAKFAST	DINNER
	LUNCH	SNACK
SAT	BREAKFAST	DINNER
	LUNCH	SNACK
SUN	BREAKFAST	DINNER
	LUNCH	SNACK

FOODS TO AVOID

_____
_____
_____
_____
_____
_____
_____
_____
_____
_____

GROCERY LIST

_____
_____
_____
_____
_____
_____
_____
_____
_____
_____
_____
_____
_____
_____
_____

Describe your typical daily diet before your colostomy surgery. Which meals or snacks did you enjoy the most?

....

....

....

....

....

....

What specific changes have you been advised to make to your diet following your colostomy? List any foods you now need to avoid or incorporate.

....

....

....

....

....

....

....

....

....

FOOD TRAKER JOURNAL

DATE:

MON	BREAKFAST		DINNER
	LUNCH		SNACK
TUE	BREAKFAST		DINNER
	LUNCH		SNACK
WED	BREAKFAST		DINNER
	LUNCH		SNACK
THUR	BREAKFAST		DINNER
	LUNCH		SNACK
FRI	BREAKFAST		DINNER
	LUNCH		SNACK
SAT	BREAKFAST		DINNER
	LUNCH		SNACK
SUN	BREAKFAST		DINNER
	LUNCH		SNACK

FOODS TO AVOID

_____
_____
_____
_____
_____
_____
_____
_____
_____

GROCERY LIST

_____
_____
_____
_____
_____
_____
_____
_____
_____
_____
_____
_____
_____
_____

How do you feel about these dietary changes? Are there any challenges you anticipate in adapting to this new diet?

....

....

....

....

....

....

What are your main nutritional goals now that you're adapting to life after colostomy surgery? (e.g., managing gas, avoiding blockages, ensuring proper hydration)

....

....

....

....

....

How do these goals compare to your dietary goals before the surgery?

....

....

....

....

FOOD TRAKER JOURNAL

DATE:

MON	BREAKFAST	DINNER
	LUNCH	SNACK
TUE	BREAKFAST	DINNER
	LUNCH	SNACK
WED	BREAKFAST	DINNER
	LUNCH	SNACK
THUR	BREAKFAST	DINNER
	LUNCH	SNACK
FRI	BREAKFAST	DINNER
	LUNCH	SNACK
SAT	BREAKFAST	DINNER
	LUNCH	SNACK
SUN	BREAKFAST	DINNER
	LUNCH	SNACK

FOODS TO AVOID

_____
_____
_____
_____
_____
_____
_____
_____

GROCERY LIST

_____
_____
_____
_____
_____
_____
_____
_____
_____
_____
_____
_____
_____

What strategies have you found effective in incorporating new foods into your diet while monitoring their impact on your colostomy?

....

....

....

....

....

....

How has your social life and dining out experiences changed since your colostomy surgery? Share a recent experience.

....

....

....

....

....

....

In what ways have you sought support or resources to help you adjust emotionally and socially to your new lifestyle?

....

....

....

....

FOOD TRAKER JOURNAL

DATE:

MON	BREAKFAST		DINNER
	LUNCH		SNACK
TUE	BREAKFAST		DINNER
	LUNCH		SNACK
WED	BREAKFAST		DINNER
	LUNCH		SNACK
THUR	BREAKFAST		DINNER
	LUNCH		SNACK
FRI	BREAKFAST		DINNER
	LUNCH		SNACK
SAT	BREAKFAST		DINNER
	LUNCH		SNACK
SUN	BREAKFAST		DINNER
	LUNCH		SNACK

FOODS TO AVOID

_____
_____
_____
_____
_____
_____
_____
_____
_____

GROCERY LIST

_____
_____
_____
_____
_____
_____
_____
_____
_____
_____
_____
_____
_____

How do you monitor your health and the effectiveness of your colostomy diet? Are there specific signs you watch for to gauge your well-being?

....

....

....

....

....

....

Describe any complications or challenges you've encountered since starting your colostomy diet. How did you address them?

....

....

....

....

....

What is the most significant lesson you've learned about managing your diet and lifestyle since your colostomy surgery?

....

....

....

....

FOOD TRAKER JOURNAL

DATE:

	BREAKFAST	DINNER
MON	LUNCH	SNACK
TUE	BREAKFAST	DINNER
	LUNCH	SNACK
WED	BREAKFAST	DINNER
	LUNCH	SNACK
THUR	BREAKFAST	DINNER
	LUNCH	SNACK
FRI	BREAKFAST	DINNER
	LUNCH	SNACK
SAT	BREAKFAST	DINNER
	LUNCH	SNACK
SUN	BREAKFAST	DINNER
	LUNCH	SNACK

FOODS TO AVOID

_____
_____
_____
_____
_____
_____
_____
_____
_____
_____

GROCERY LIST

_____
_____
_____
_____
_____
_____
_____
_____
_____
_____
_____
_____
_____
_____
_____

Identify one or two areas where you feel you need more information or support regarding your colostomy diet. How do you plan to seek out this information?

....

....

....

....

....

....

....

....

....

....

....

How do you envision your diet and lifestyle continuing to evolve in the future? Set one long-term goal related to your colostomy management.

....

....

....

FOOD TRAKER JOURNAL

DATE:

		BREAKFAST	DINNER
MON		LUNCH	SNACK
TUE		BREAKFAST	DINNER
		LUNCH	SNACK
WED		BREAKFAST	DINNER
		LUNCH	SNACK
THUR		BREAKFAST	DINNER
		LUNCH	SNACK
FRI		BREAKFAST	DINNER
		LUNCH	SNACK
SAT		BREAKFAST	DINNER
		LUNCH	SNACK
SUN		BREAKFAST	DINNER
		LUNCH	SNACK

FOODS TO AVOID

_____
_____
_____
_____
_____
_____
_____
_____
_____

GROCERY LIST

_____
_____
_____
_____
_____
_____
_____
_____
_____
_____
_____
_____
_____
_____

FOOD TRAKER JOURNAL

DATE:

			FOODS TO AVOID
MON	BREAKFAST	DINNER	_____
	LUNCH	SNACK	_____
TUE	BREAKFAST	DINNER	_____
	LUNCH	SNACK	_____
WED	BREAKFAST	DINNER	_____
	LUNCH	SNACK	**GROCERY LIST**
THUR	BREAKFAST	DINNER	_____
	LUNCH	SNACK	_____
FRI	BREAKFAST	DINNER	_____
	LUNCH	SNACK	_____
SAT	BREAKFAST	DINNER	_____
	LUNCH	SNACK	_____
SUN	BREAKFAST	DINNER	_____
	LUNCH	SNACK	_____

FOOD TRAKER JOURNAL

DATE: _____

MON	BREAKFAST	DINNER
	LUNCH	SNACK
TUE	BREAKFAST	DINNER
	LUNCH	SNACK
WED	BREAKFAST	DINNER
	LUNCH	SNACK
THUR	BREAKFAST	DINNER
	LUNCH	SNACK
FRI	BREAKFAST	DINNER
	LUNCH	SNACK
SAT	BREAKFAST	DINNER
	LUNCH	SNACK
SUN	BREAKFAST	DINNER
	LUNCH	SNACK

FOODS TO AVOID
_____
_____
_____
_____
_____
_____
_____
_____
_____

GROCERY LIST
_____
_____
_____
_____
_____
_____
_____
_____
_____
_____
_____
_____
_____
_____
_____

FOOD TRAKER JOURNAL

DATE:

MON	BREAKFAST	DINNER
	LUNCH	SNACK
TUE	BREAKFAST	DINNER
	LUNCH	SNACK
WED	BREAKFAST	DINNER
	LUNCH	SNACK
THUR	BREAKFAST	DINNER
	LUNCH	SNACK
FRI	BREAKFAST	DINNER
	LUNCH	SNACK
SAT	BREAKFAST	DINNER
	LUNCH	SNACK
SUN	BREAKFAST	DINNER
	LUNCH	SNACK

FOODS TO AVOID

_____
_____
_____
_____
_____
_____
_____
_____
_____

GROCERY LIST

_____
_____
_____
_____
_____
_____
_____
_____
_____
_____
_____
_____
_____
_____

FOOD TRAKER JOURNAL

DATE:

MON	BREAKFAST	DINNER	
	LUNCH	SNACK	
TUE	BREAKFAST	DINNER	
	LUNCH	SNACK	
WED	BREAKFAST	DINNER	
	LUNCH	SNACK	
THUR	BREAKFAST	DINNER	
	LUNCH	SNACK	
FRI	BREAKFAST	DINNER	
	LUNCH	SNACK	
SAT	BREAKFAST	DINNER	
	LUNCH	SNACK	
SUN	BREAKFAST	DINNER	
	LUNCH	SNACK	

FOODS TO AVOID
_____
_____
_____
_____
_____
_____
_____
_____
_____
_____

GROCERY LIST
_____
_____
_____
_____
_____
_____
_____
_____
_____
_____
_____
_____
_____
_____
_____
_____
_____

FOOD TRAKER JOURNAL

DATE:

MON	BREAKFAST	DINNER
	LUNCH	SNACK
TUE	BREAKFAST	DINNER
	LUNCH	SNACK
WED	BREAKFAST	DINNER
	LUNCH	SNACK
THUR	BREAKFAST	DINNER
	LUNCH	SNACK
FRI	BREAKFAST	DINNER
	LUNCH	SNACK
SAT	BREAKFAST	DINNER
	LUNCH	SNACK
SUN	BREAKFAST	DINNER
	LUNCH	SNACK

FOODS TO AVOID

GROCERY LIST

Scan the QR code below to get a surprise bonus!

If you would love to have a one-on-one consultation session with Dr. Kelly Haaland, kindly reach out to us at kellyhaaland2@gmail.com.

www.ingramcontent.com/pod-product-compliance
Lightning Source LLC
Chambersburg PA
CBHW062106220526
45471CB00010B/3621